☙ ☙

GEORGE LEA HARPER, JR., is on disability leave from his position as professor of religion at Pembroke State University, Pembroke, North Carolina. An ordained United Methodist minister, he has published articles in *The Christian Century* and in *Religion and Intellectual Life*.

Living with Dying

Finding Meaning in Chronic Illness

George Lea Harper, Jr.

WILLIAM B. EERDMANS PUBLISHING COMPANY

GRAND RAPIDS, MICHIGAN

Library of Congress Cataloging-in-Publication Data

Harper, George Lea, 1945-
    Living with dying : finding meaning in chronic illness /
George Lea Harper, Jr.
        p.   cm.
    ISBN 0-8028-0631-7 (pbk.)
    1. Chronic diseases — Religious aspects — Christianity.
2. Cancer — Religious aspects — Christianity.   I. Title.
RC108.H37   1992
362.1'96994 — dc20   92-212
                                                          CIP

Unless otherwise noted, Scripture quotations are from the Revised
Standard Version of the Bible, copyrighted 1946, 1952 © 1971,
1973 by the Division of Christian Education of the National Coun-
cil of the Churches of Christ in the U.S.A., and used by permission.

Contents

Foreword ────────────────

GEORGE LEA HARPER IS DYING. Of course, so am I. We're both terminal. The difference between George Lea Harper and me is that he knows he's dying whereas I don't. He has stood on the cliff, stooped over, and peered into the dark abyss. He has heard the owl call his name.

So George Lea Harper has much to tell us. On a day like today when I'm feeling fine, I need to hear the truthful testimony which he has achieved by facing his own finitude. Tomorrow, when I may not be feeling so fine and it is my turn to walk that lonely path toward Death, I will need to hear his hopeful word that I do not walk that path alone.

This is a book which displays a rare but utterly Christian virtue. It combines both truth and hope. Harper is a realist. What he describes will evoke repeated nods of recognition in anyone who has lived with chronic illness. With quiet, confident eloquence, George Lea Harper speaks of these matters which the rest of us find tough to put into words. From envy of normal neighbors to confessions of impatience, to a wonderful excursus on "sick humor," George Lea Harper helps us to find meaning in an event which too often destroys and defies meaning. This book is therefore an act of faith, an affirmation that even in our darkest days, God graciously gives us light. These short meditations will provide hours of reflection. This is the book one could give to a friend who is now dealing with dying. The book says for us what we wish we could say to that friend. It can be read alone or in a group. Whether it is read during an acute crisis of dying, or as a part of preparing (as are we all) for Death to tap us on the shoulder and bid us to follow, this book will change you.

John Wesley, father of my Methodism, once bragged of his Methodists, "Our people die well." For Wesley, the supreme compliment to the quality of their lives was the dignified defiance of their dying.

God grant that through *Living with Dying,* the same might be said for us.

William H. Willimon
Dean of the Chapel and Professor
of Christian Ministry
Duke University

Acknowledgments ————————————

THE WRITER OF ANY BOOK, I believe, accumulates enormous debts which can never be adequately acknowledged, let alone repaid. Because of my illness, I have incurred more debts than most authors. Furthermore, since my writing of this book turns upon my own experiences in living with dying, all of those people who have assisted me during recent years have become part of the supporting cast. I thank them all, but must say additional words about the following persons.

For "hands-on" care across months and months of treatment, I thank the staff members of the following facilities: Medical Hematology/Oncology Clinic and Jordan Ward, Duke University Medical Center (Durham, NC); Short Stay Center, Cape Fear Valley Medical Center (Fayetteville,

NC); Station 75, Lymphoma/Myeloma/Bone Marrow Transplant, M.D. Anderson Cancer Center (Houston, TX); Phase One Clinic, Cancer Therapy and Research Center (San Antonio, TX). They may not know it, but about seventy-five percent of this book was written on yellow legal pads during treatment in their facilities.

For humane guidance in evaluation and therapy, I thank these medical doctors who have treated me across the past six years: Wayne Brenckman, Rueben N. Rivers, Fredrick Hagemeister, Joseph O. Moore, and Charles F. LeMaistre.

For welcome diversion, recreation, and smiles during therapy, I thank the Oncology Recreation Therapy volunteers, and for uplifting counsel, the Cancer Patient Support Program, both at Duke University Medical Center.

Outside the clinics and hospitals, my family and I have been assisted by many people. For encouragement and support "on the job" before I took disability leave — and since — I thank Dr. Robert K. Gustafson and Dr. Charles R. Jenkins of Pembroke State University (Pembroke, NC). For prayers, child care, and other "life support," my family and I thank the members of these United Methodist churches: Fellowship (Hamlet, NC), St. Matthew's (Fayetteville, NC), and Epworth (Durham, NC). For becoming "substitute parents," my wife and I thank Birgit and Peter Sauer, our former neighbors in Fayetteville. They fed, chauffered, and assisted our sons with school projects while I was hospitalized away from home. For housing and hospitality my gratitude goes to Dr. and Mrs. Dennis M. Campbell and Mr. and Mrs. Carl Fick. For special services I thank Dr. Thomas E. Harper and family. Tom is brother, translator of medical "jargon," provider of housing, and friend.

As I completed work on the manuscript of this book, still others assisted me. For reading parts of the manuscript and aiding me in contacting possible publishers, my thanks go to Dr. and Mrs. Robert L. Wilson and to Dr. William H. Willimon. A special word of gratitude also goes to Dr. Willimon for agreeing to write the Foreword. For their enthusiastic acceptance of my manuscript and for their guidance in publication, I thank the staff of William B. Eerdmans Publishing Company, particularly Jennifer Hoffman, who edited the book.

In the pages which follow I will often reflect upon biblical texts. I will mention one here, at the end of my acknowledgments. John's Gospel records the story in which Jesus turns water into wine — his first miracle in this Gospel. After the supply of wine gives out and Jesus miraculously provides more, the steward of the feast declares to the bridegroom, "You have kept the good wine until now" (2:10). The analogy to my situation isn't perfect, but I have saved my greatest thanks until last. My wife Ruth first urged me to record my reflections upon living with dying. As I began a seven-week series of every-other-day treatments for a lung infection, she encouraged me to use my time to write down what I was thinking. While I intended to write several articles, she believed that a book would emerge. She nursed me through chemotherapy and surgery, pastored local churches, and mothered our two sons. Somewhere in that schedule she found time to critique my developing manuscript, to type chapters, and to urge me to keep writing. Without Ruth I probably would not have lived this long with cancer. Without Ruth, surely there would have been no book. To her I dedicate these pages.

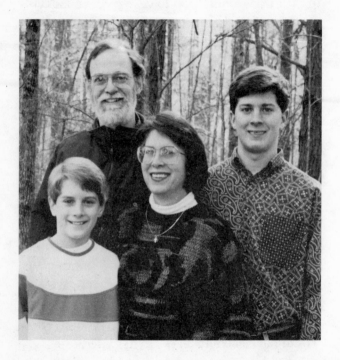

With my son Nathan, wife Ruth, and son Eric

Introduction

WITH MANY OTHERS I have shared a growing interest in issues of life, death, and the role of faith in recent years. As an ordained minister (in the United Methodist Church) and a former college teacher of religion, my own journey into these issues has been guided by the compass of my Christian faith. But another element has also pressed me onward: I am a man who has cancer. For more than six years now, this reality has shaped my life, my work, and my faith.

My cancer has developed with many faces. At first, it was a distant though menacing threat. I did not feel ill and received no treatment. Then came months of chemotherapy, with the usual side effects of nausea and hair loss. Accompanying chemotherapy were bouts of life-threatening pneumonia. The name of my disease has also changed. During four months in early 1985 doctors were uncertain what to call my illness. Then I was told that I had chronic lymphocytic leukemia; later this was relabeled "small cell lymphoma." By whatever name, my disease is systemic. At least in my case, this cancer has no viable cure. So far I have undergone eight different kinds of chemotherapy or experimental treatments plus one major surgery. In recent years my life has become a conscious process of "living with dying."

I share this personal background not to evoke sympathy — I don't like pity and would emphasize that as I write I am still *living* with dying. But this background is the necessary foundation for the chapters which follow. They are a record of wrestlings with life, death, and hope. They combine my encounters and those of my family with cancer, with the medical community, with each other, and with our faith.

During this familial journey spanning more than six years, we have discovered numerous factual guides to cancer and many manuals offering psychological help. But we have found few practical resources which examine the struggle of living with cancer through the eyes of Christian faith. In talking with pastors and church members, cancer patients and their families, I have learned that others also seek such materials. I have also discovered that the task of living with a major chronic illness has been shared by a growing number of persons in recent years. Many of us who are cancer, heart, or kidney patients today would not have survived so long even ten years ago. Major advances in diagnosis and treatment have increased our life spans. A recent report found that the average survival rate after initial diagnosis of cancer is now almost two-and-one-half years.

With increased life span, however, comes a major challenge: how do you live with a disease which, in all probability, will eventually kill you? How does the individual, and his or her family, cope with the ups and downs of treatments? With complexities of decision-making about what to do next? With maintaining routine and some semblance of "normalcy" in family relations? With agonizing questions about God and one's faith? These reflections have been developed to address such questions, for myself and for others. Throughout, I have tried to provide a dialogue between biblical material and the everyday experiences of one man (and his family) with cancer. While cancer is the primary illness of reference, much of the discussion will apply to other chronic illnesses as well.

The unifying theme of this book, then, will be the role of Christian faith in the lives of those who are living with dying. The emphasis will not be upon ready answers but upon the struggle to discover, for each new day, the vitality, direction, and hope which faith can bring. My prayer for these chapters is that they may assist others who live with dying — whether as patients, family members, pastors, or friends.

I make no assumption that our experiences are exactly the same. Still, I hope those who read these reflections will find in them some insights both into how chronic illness — cancer in particular — attacks life and into how faith can function as a counterthrust of hope and healing. With you I share the peaks and valleys of this different and difficult existence. With you I also share the moments of victory of the human spirit which so many of our "healthy" acquaintances miss. And perhaps with you I can share a growing kinship with the divine spirit — a kinship nurtured as we travel down a road of hardship we would not choose, but where we can finally triumph.

Facing Death ————————————————

OUR SOCIETY FEARS DEATH. We seek to distance ourselves from it and to avoid it at all costs. We try to convince ourselves that if we eat right and exercise, we can all live to be eighty and then die in our sleep. We also seek to shield our children from death. I recall one woman who told me of the difficulty she had had as a child coping with the accidental death of her pet dog. She wanted to spare her daughter the same anguish, so she would not allow her to have any pets. Avoid pets and perhaps we can avoid death.

Even the church sometimes cooperates in this avoidance behavior. Bishop Howard E. Wennes of the Grand Canyon Synod, Evangelical Lutheran Church in America, recently declared: "We need to bring the reality of death back into the sanctuary and onto the agendas of people's lives."*

Fearing my own death, I followed society's lead for years. I jogged, ate right, and had regular physical checkups. Still, at age forty I contracted cancer. I had feared a heart attack, but cancer snuck up on me! Wrestling with my cancer has forced me to confront my own mortality. Unavoidably we all die. I am no different from anyone else in this way, though my timetable may be shorter than some. Sitting in the local hospital's short-stay center recently, I overheard this conversation. Patient: "You think I'm going to make it?" Doctor: "You're going to make it. I don't know how long. I don't know for myself either. I don't know the answer to those questions." A wise physician, this one, who admits even his own mortality!

Our deaths are inevitable. But being forced to confront my own, I have come to a surprising realization: facing my own death has brought me a strange new sense of freedom. I cannot avoid dying. Even my best efforts and those of the best doctors cannot change this fact. But having accepted it, I find that I have become more relaxed

* *United Methodist Reporter,* 16 June 1989.

about living my life during the time that remains. The author of Hebrews declares that Jesus became human "that through death he might . . . deliver all those who through fear of death were subject to lifelong bondage" (2:14-15). Even in life, we become prisoners of death through our fear of it and our efforts to avoid it. Death can paralyze us, preventing us from living fully long before we draw our last breath. We need deliverance.

What I will call a "theology of surrender" operates here. It is through surrendering to God's will that I have begun to overcome my fear of death. "Perfect love casts out fear" (1 John 4:18). I am coming to trust God's will for my life and death. The prayer of Stanley Kresge, shared with me by Dr. William K. Quick, has become my own: "Thy will, O Lord, nothing more, nothing less, nothing else, thy will." This brief prayer echoed in my mind as I faced lung surgery, bringing with it a sense of inner peace. I am aware that confronting death in this way does not alter its eventual certainty, nor does it ward off pain and suffering. But it can at least lessen the fear of pain and death which paralyzes us.

> The people who walked in darkness
>   have seen a great light;

those who dwelt in a land of deep darkness,
    on them has light shined.

(Isa. 9:2)

But surrendering our lives to God in this way is very difficult. We struggle to understand how our deaths could be part of God's plan. The story of Peter can be helpful to us here. Before his crucifixion, Jesus sought to prepare his disciples for the events to come:

> And he began to teach them that the Son of man must suffer many things, and be rejected by the elders and the chief priests and the scribes, and be killed, and after three days rise again. And he said this plainly. And Peter took him, and began to rebuke him. But turning and seeing his disciples, he rebuked Peter . . . (Mark 8:31-33)

Like us, Peter cannot see how death could be part of God's plan. He mistakenly argues for Christ's earthly life and is rebuked for his failure to understand. Christ then goes even further, saying that Peter himself cannot avoid death: "For whoever would save his life will lose it; and whoever loses his life for my sake and the gospel's will save it" (Mark 8:35). Still Peter does not understand; later his fear of death leads him to deny Christ three times (Mark 14:66-72). But Peter's story does not end there. His faith grew and he became able to confront his fear as a faithful disciple, courageously preaching the gospel wherever he went. According to tradition, Peter was eventually crucified for his faith, upside down, in Rome.

We in the contemporary church can learn from Peter. Like him, we fear death — sometimes even to the extent of denying Jesus. We must learn to face the reality of death, accepting death as an inevitable part of our life, and surrendering both to God. Perhaps Bishop Wennes' proposal could help: "Why not have funerals on Sunday morning? Funerals won't disturb our worship. They will help to define our message. In Christ we have God's answer to death."*

* Ibid.

Living out of Control ──────────

LIVING YEAR IN AND YEAR OUT with chronic illness changes your worldview. Normal routines and assumptions crumble under the weight of countless tests and protracted treatment. One's life — personal, family, and professional — is turned upside down. For myself and for my family, coping with the loss of control has been one of the most difficult adjustments we've had to make.

From childhood on in our society we learn to plan ahead. "The early bird gets the worm," we are told. We start early in planning for our children and in mapping our careers. Our vacations and even our retirements are plotted in advance. Individual retirement accounts and company benefit plans allow us to project comfortable "golden years." When chronic illness impinges, however, our ability to plan ahead diminishes dramatically. Over the six years since I was diagnosed with cancer (now identified as lymphoma), our family's ability to plan ahead has eroded steadily. Arranging for a summer vacation, for example, becomes a "shot in the dark," since we cannot accurately predict when I will be receiving more chemotherapy or when I may need to be hospitalized for infection. Every commitment is prefaced with *If* . . . Often we feel our lives are out of control.

This predicament is often difficult for others to understand. Two years ago my five brothers and sisters began planning a family reunion. We were to meet in North Carolina over Memorial Day weekend, converging from Ohio, Texas, Florida, and points in between. Two weeks before Memorial Day, however, I was hospitalized in Houston, Texas, undergoing treatment for a fungal infection. Would I make the reunion? No one knew. Finally it was canceled, one week beforehand. On the chosen weekend I was back home, still undergoing every-other-day treatments, but feeling much better. The reunion was rescheduled, with no assurances for next time.

After months of such uncertainty, my wife

and I found ourselves yearning for our neighbors' existence. Theirs are predictable lives. To work at 7:30, home by 5:00. He plays golf on Saturday, she suns. Summer Caribbean cruises are routine. Their lives are smooth, planned — some might say boring. We sometimes covet a portion of their routine for ourselves. We would even welcome boredom. The scheduled existence which we used to accept and sometimes complain about is gone. Even attending church together, with dinner out afterward, can't be taken for granted.

Responding theologically to my illness and our loss of control has been difficult. Hope is important, but what I call a theology of surrender has become most meaningful. Like St. Paul, we see through the glass only darkly. So often I have prayed with Jesus, "If thou art willing, remove this cup from me; nevertheless not my will, but thine, be done" (Luke 22:42). In uttering this prayer I am confessing that I don't know how my illness will progress. I'm still unable to plan ahead. But it helps me to become increasingly willing to leave my future up to God.

At one level this surrender reflects the simple gospel I learned in childhood. It is one of those basic truths which Robert Fulghum probably learned in kindergarten.* In the words of the old hymn, "all to Jesus I surrender, all to Him I freely give."** This surrender cannot be just a means to a selfish end — even that of healing. It is not a bargaining with God in which I say, "Heal me and I will serve you better." But neither is it simple resignation in which hope has died. It is surrender in trust. In this surrender one relinquishes control to God.

Such surrender does not come easily, though. It means relinquishing my desire to plan ahead and to know the future with certainty. It goes against all my natural impulses — but it is faithful. Like Moses at the burning bush, I sometimes try to escape my need to surrender to God; I want to keep some semblance of control. But also like Moses, I seem unable to escape. I need God to guide me on my journey through the wilderness because I do not know the route. I don't always see the cloud by day or pillar of fire by night (Exod. 13:21), but I know the Lord is with me — even when I doubt. I still often feel out of control and struggle with my eroded ability to

* See Fulghum's book *All I Really Need to Know I Learned in Kindergarten* (Random House, 1988).
** *Cokesbury Worship Hymnal,* no. 148.

make plans, but with God's help I can learn to pray with Jesus, "Father, into thy hands I commit my spirit!" (Luke 23:46).

Living Past, Vital Present, Unknown Future ――――

ONE'S PERSPECTIVE UPON TIME changes through the confrontation with cancer. Consider the future. Before my illness the future was a horizon of hope. True, my options were shrinking a bit as I entered middle age, but the future was still open-ended. Possibilities for development in my job, for relationships with my children, and for personal growth seemed broad if not limitless. Since my diagnosis with cancer, however, my future has been clouded. I used to take the arrival of a new day for granted; now each new day is a gift. My younger son asked in October several years ago if I would live until Christmas. How could I respond? Shortly afterward I asked my doctor about my prognosis. How long could I expect to live? He didn't know, he said. But when pressed he continued, "Barring complications, you should be here this Christmas. Next Christmas is another matter."

This dramatic change in my perspective on the future has also reshaped my attitude toward the past. Probably because of my age (mid-forties), and surely because of my illness, I have reflected deeply upon my past. It has become a storehouse of memories to which I can readily return as my future shrinks. Friendships and memories from college years are renewed through reunions and letters. Childhood vacations and incidents are relived with parents, brothers, and sisters. Nostalgic visits to former homes take on new significance. My past expands as my future contracts.

The present has also taken on a new significance. No longer is it simply the gateway to the future, a means toward some future end. Rather, the present — along with memories of the past — is all that I have. This shift in orientation has underscored the importance of my stewardship of the present. Jesus' parable of the talents (Matt. 25:14-30), which focuses on the believer's current responsibilities, takes on new meaning for the person who is chronically ill. The wise servants in the parable, not knowing when the master will return, act prudently in the present to invest the resources allotted to them. Matthew even notes that the man receiving five talents left "at once and traded with them; and he made five talents more" (v. 16). Living responsibly in the present is thus important for Jesus, and it has new significance for me.

But for others who are not themselves chronically ill, the present does not have quite the same urgency. My wife and children are forced to plan ahead. Ruth has conference sessions to attend and church meetings to oversee. My sons have to plan ahead for school commitments and church day-camp. For them the future is not so clouded. Their lives require planning for the future and less concern about the past. These different perspectives entail some tension and even conflict within the family. Ruth and the boys must plan ahead; I cannot. Our family life thus becomes a balancing act, with a great need for mutual understanding. I share in making plans for trips, the boys' programs, etc., however tentatively. They try to live fully in the present, not postponing everything until later.

This living between past and future is a constant roller coaster ride in which the passengers are blindfolded, unable to see the approaching curves or drops. Gradually one adjusts. But are there any grounds for hope? How many times during my illness have we heard doctors assure us that this will be *the* treatment. "We'll get a lot of mileage out of this drug!" one said. Two months later I was in the hospital with cancer infiltrating my right lung. After a bronchoscopy, we were told that the wonder drug would have to be stopped and strong conventional chemotherapy begun. Since then we have heard again that I might be a candidate for another experimental treatment.

What does one hope for, when the future is so clouded? Each new promise seems to carry its companion disappointment. I recall the words of a widow whose husband suffered from the same form of cancer that I suffer from. A revival meeting was held at his church. At the close of the service the preacher asked all those who wanted prayers for healing to come forward. Her husband remained seated in the pew. Later, at home, she asked him why. "I can't handle getting my hopes up again," he said. "I don't think I could handle the disappointment. At least I've adjusted to where I am." I can understand his reluctance. The roller coaster ride of hope and disappointment is draining. One grows tired of the struggle.

Is hope then dead for the chronically ill? Gradually I have realized that, while I cannot trust in the future itself, I can trust the God of the future. It is not I who "keep [my] going out and [my] coming in from this time forth and for evermore" (Ps. 121:8). The future of Jesus as he faced the cross also looked dismal. But through faith in his Father, Jesus endured the present and won a new dimension of life. I don't know what my future holds. But through faith in God I can aspire to share this new life with Christ. I don't know its nature, but I do have the example of Jesus and can strive to follow him. "I came that they may have life, and have it abundantly" (John 10:10).

Wrestling with
the Angel of Illness ──────────

IN POPULAR THINKING, enduring illness and suffering is often equated with "bearing one's cross." Since the cross is the central symbol of Christian faith, I have mulled over this perspective. "If any man would come after me, let him deny himself and take up his cross and follow me" (Mark 8:34). How does the cross which Jesus mentions here relate to illness, particularly chronic illness?

Living with suffering is not in itself bearing one's cross. No one chooses the suffering of chronic illness. The crossbearing related to illness emerges in one's *response* to one's condition. One can choose to accept the challenges brought by suffering. This choice need not imply ready acquiescence or passive resignation. As St. Paul told the Corinthians, he prayed vigorously for removal of his thorn in the flesh, yet he continued to suffer (2 Cor. 12:7-9).

For many of us, wrestling with our illness relates to the experiences of the Old Testament figure Jacob. Like us, Jacob does all within his power to control his situation. Awaiting his encounter with his brother Esau, whom he had tricked out of his birthright, he divides his company into two parts, hoping that at least one group will survive if Esau attacks. He also prays to God, recounting God's past promises, and he sends gifts to Esau (Gen. 32:7-13). Living with chronic illness, we too struggle for control. We seek new treatments and different doctors. We bargain with God, even citing Jesus' words from Scripture, as if to remind God of his promises:

Ask, and it will be given you . . . (Matt. 7:7)

Therefore I tell you, whatever you ask in prayer, believe that you have received it, and it will be yours. (Mark 11:24)

If you abide in me, and my words abide in you, ask whatever you will, and it shall be done for you. (John 15:7)

[21]

Help us out of this mess, Lord, and we will surely glorify you!

Despite our best efforts, when we engage in our solitary wrestling with illness, we do not emerge unscathed. We are *marked* persons, even if we survive. The night before he was to meet Esau, Jacob engaged in a wrestling match with an "angel" at the Jabbok ford. When the angel did not overcome Jacob, "he touched the hollow of his thigh; and Jacob's thigh was put out of joint." Jacob limped as he left his adversary. Israelite tradition commemorates his encounter by proscribing the eating of sinew from the hip of animals (Gen. 32:22-32). We who struggle with chronic illness are also marked for life. Our illness affects, among other things, the way we do theology. Wrestling with the angel of our illness recasts our thinking about our faith.

At the heart of this recasting is our encounter with God. We meet God, indeed wrestle with God, as we confront our illness. As I mentioned earlier, more than resignation occurs here. We bargain and protest, seeking control. We are marked in the struggle. For we struggle not just with the illness itself but also with our Creator. (The Israelite tradition interprets Jacob's new name "Israel," given to him by the angel, as "he who strives with God" [Gen. 32:28].) Our illness becomes the *occasion* for our wrestling with God; our illness is our Jabbok ford.

This wrestling also reminds us of Job's encounter with God. Job was in the throes of illness when he wrestled with God. In his case, even more than Jacob's, the theological dimension is explicit:

> Then the LORD answered Job out of
> the whirlwind:
> "Who is this that darkens counsel
> by words without knowledge?
> Gird up your loins like a man,
> I will question you, and you shall
> declare to me."
>
> (Job 38:1-3)

Like Jacob, Job struggles with God and is changed in the process:

> I had heard of thee by the hearing of the ear,
> but now my eye sees thee;
> therefore I despise myself,
> and repent in dust and ashes.
>
> (42:5-6)

[23]

Illness thus becomes the occasion for an encounter with God. Out of the wrestling comes a new relationship.

One dimension of Job's experience is particularly significant for those wrestling with chronic illness: Job does not receive an answer to all the "Why?" questions he has hurled at God. In the end Job simply says, "I have uttered what I did not understand . . ." (42:3). Instead of getting answers, Job — like Jacob — meets God face-to-face. A new personal relationship replaces a quest for understanding.

Thus the suffering of chronic illness may become the avenue for new encounters with God. Illness is not something we seek or volunteer for. But when we are faced with disease, we can respond by wrestling with God. Rather than betraying the Creator, this wrestling can bring us to an invigorated relationship with God, even if it does not yield answers to all our questions. "Taking up our cross" thus involves confronting our illnesses head on, not dodging the hard questions. God can "take it," as the cases of Job and Jacob illustrate. Through this confrontation we take up our crosses and follow Christ.

Samson Revisited:
Long Hair, No Hair ──────────

WHILE IN SEMINARY I let my hair grow long. I
kept it that way most of the time until my first
course of chemotherapy. Then I didn't have to
cut it. It fell out on its own! This experience of
losing my hair during treatment was traumatic
for me, as it is for many people. Why?

Reflecting upon this question, I have discovered several reasons. My hair had become,
over two decades, part of my identity. A member
of the rock musical "Hair" generation, I let my
hair grow almost shoulder length during my
early twenties. When the photographer took my
picture for the pictorial lineup of former as-
sociate pastors at the first church I served, he
asked to take extra shots. He thought I looked

[25]

like a biblical prophet with my long hair and beard! One parishioner told me when I arrived at the church that he had three goals for me to accomplish while I was there: to cut my hair, to get married, and to gain weight. (None of the three happened during that year.) At another church I finally cut my beard and trimmed my hair because of objections from some members.

Part of my reason for having long hair, I recognize, was protest. From seminary days on, I saw many problems with the "establishment," inside and outside the church. By wearing my hair long, I was not "selling out" completely. My long hair was a visible symbol that I was "different."

But when chemo began, the long hair went — not voluntarily! I remember the first time this happened, while it was still long. With brushing my hair would come out in clumps. My wife, who says she enjoyed playing with my curls, once reached up to touch one, and it came out in her hand. Hot oil treatments did little to slow the process. We collected the lost hair in a plastic bag.

Often these experiences of losing my hair have made me think of the story of Samson in the book of Judges. As a Nazirite, Samson was instructed by God not to cut his hair (Judg. 13:5). While it was long, he retained his strength. But when he finally surrendered to Delilah's nagging and his hair was cut, he lost his power. The spirit of God departed from him (16:4-20). I don't directly connect the spirit of God in my own life with hair, but the Samson saga is significant for me.

Looking back, I now see that when my hair began to come out, I lost part of my identity. Samson's hair marked him as a Nazirite; mine gave me a sense that I was "my own man," that I didn't subscribe to all social customs. When I was preparing for ordination in the Methodist Church (not then United Methodist), one pastor asked me, "How can you stand transparent before the cross with a beard?" As I sought to explain, I understood that following Christ sometimes placed one at odds with cultural patterns. My own hair length and beard were to me symbols of my position. In my mind, they helped identify who I was.

When my hair and beard began to fall out, however, I lost the symbols of my identity. Like Samson, I took on a new role. He became a victim; I became a patient — and I looked like an elderly man. The change came suddenly for both of us. Delilah's trim took only minutes. Most of my hair came out in several days, particularly when washed or brushed. With less and less hair each day, I assumed that look which marks people on chemotherapy: very thin, stringy hair, with mostly scalp showing. Even then I clung to my old self, not shaving my head or what was left of my beard. The first time this happened (so far, my hair has come out six times), my sons were understandably embarrassed to be seen with me. One nurse mistook my wife for my daughter. And while visiting my brother's church I was asked, "Are you Tom's father?" Losing one's usual identity is difficult enough. Assuming the new identity of patient or older parent in the eyes of the world compounds the problem.

With this change in appearance came a new vulnerability. Samson was blinded and bound in chains (Judg. 16:21). I felt a sense of being exposed, of being naked before the world. Curious stares of people on the street underscored the change. (My brother insightfully observed that space creatures in the movies are usually bald and are called "aliens"!) Several acquaintances at work did not even recognize me. But a real, physical vulnerability was also present. Outside in the sun, my head would burn if I didn't wear a cap. During the winter I needed a hat to keep my head warm. Sometimes I even wore it inside, in church, when the ceiling fans blew directly on me. Here physical comfort overrode etiquette and tradition.

My experiences with hair don't end here, however. When a series of chemotherapy treatments ends, my hair returns. Like Samson, I recover part of my old self, though I too have been changed by the experience. My hair is thinner now, even when not receiving treatment. I wear it shorter, but still with the beard. Chameleon-like, I change from almost no hair to hairy again. The change reflects my life itself, the ups and downs of living with cancer. Illness leaves its mark, but the effort to cling to health and to choose my identity continues. No hair, long hair — Samson would understand!

Negative Leaven,
Sour Family Relationships

IN DESCRIBING THE KINGDOM OF HEAVEN, Jesus at one point compares it to leaven. A woman takes a tiny bit of leaven and stirs it into three measures of flour. Eventually all the flour is leavened by this small addition (Matt. 13:33). During the six years since I was diagnosed with cancer, my illness has worked as a negative leaven in our family life. At first the intrusions were small enough: visits to the oncologist every several months, with accompanying tests. But as treatments began, the impact on our family became greater. Now the chemotherapy caused me to miss work a week at a time. My wife was away from our sons more as she spent increasing amounts of time with me at the hospital. My illness became real and unavoidable to everyone when I returned home with nausea and as I began to lose my hair.

After I was referred to an out-of-state cancer center, the situation became even worse. I was now gone two or three weeks at a time, never knowing as I left when I would return. Nor did I know whether I would receive treatment or surgery for which my wife would want to be present. She would await news by telephone, uncertain what to expect.

We have discovered, therefore, that my cancer, as a chronic illness, infects the whole family. Cancer strikes at the fabric of our family relationships. In a sense, all of the family members become disabled. My wife in particular has experienced this reality. As she says, she is pulled in three directions: by her job as parish pastor, by our sons, and by me. The needs in the local church go on, whether I am ill or not. Members are gracious, but they too experience illness and pain which require ministry. Programs must be planned and meetings conducted. All of this requires full-time effort, but Ruth is torn among divided loyalties. Weeks spent with me while I'm hospitalized mean that her ministry suffers. In fact, as she aptly puts it, my illness has been as disabling for her in her work as it has been for me in mine.

Ruth also devotes much time and energy to our two sons. When I am away, full responsibility for their care falls upon her. Even more than usual she becomes chauffeur, cook, and caregiver. But time spent with them is time spent away from church work. And whether with the boys or working at the church, she worries about me. My illness has violently disrupted her life as mother, pastor, and wife. No matter how hard she tries, she cannot do enough for any of her three "constituencies." She too is disabled by my cancer, to a degree that few recognize.

Our two sons are also affected. Nathan, our eleven-year-old, prays every night for my healing. When I am hospitalized his mind wanders and his school work suffers. Recently he asked his mother, "Where will we live if Daddy dies?" Our best efforts to sustain his normal schedule cannot protect him from the reality of my disease. Nor do we want to hide the truth from him. For Eric, our sixteen-year-old, fears are somewhat different. He doesn't talk much about my cancer, but he does inquire how I am doing and asks if my lymphoma can be inherited. For weeks on end, both boys live with their father a thousand miles away, undergoing strange treatments with unknown results. Grandparents, church members, and neighbors provide care, food, and transportation. But life remains confused. St. Paul could not have described our situation better: "If one member suffers, all suffer together" (1 Cor. 12:26).

Whether in the church as the body of Christ or in the family as a subunit of that body, the illness of one member can radically affect the other members. As individuals and as the whole body, they suffer. Where two have become one flesh, the disability of one partner is shared by the other. Life cannot go on as usual for anyone in the family unit. The story of Saul and his son Jonathan in the Old Testament illustrates how one father's illness affects his son. Plagued by mental instability, Saul is jealous of the praise given to his young courtier David. When Jonathan seeks to intervene on David's behalf, Saul hurls a spear at his own son, seeking to kill him (1 Sam. 20:30-34). Jonathan helps David to escape (20:35-42), but he also remains loyal to his father. Later Jonathan dies in his father's ill-fated battle with the Philistines (31:2).

"If one member suffers, all suffer together," Paul said in his first letter to the Corinthians.

And in his second letter to the church at Corinth he offers other words that may speak to us in our dilemma:

> But we have this treasure in earthen vessels, to show that the transcendent power belongs to God and not to us. We are afflicted in every way, but not crushed; perplexed, but not driven to despair; persecuted, but not forsaken; struck down, but not destroyed; always carrying in the body the death of Jesus, so that the life of Jesus may also be manifested in our bodies. (2 Cor. 4:7-10)

My cancer has been a radical reminder that our love as husband, wife, and children is contained in earthen vessels. These vessels break and eventually return to dust. Sometimes we have celebrated our love and relationships as though they were independent of God. We can do that no longer. The earthly love we share, no matter how strong, can be broken. Cancer comes between us. "Transcendent power belongs to God and not to us." Paul speaks powerfully to our situation in the verses that follow this assertion. He is realistic without being pessimistic. Although our circumstances differ from his, we too feel afflicted, perplexed, persecuted, struck down.

Sometimes we are on the verge of despair and feel almost forsaken, but Paul's words elsewhere draw us back from the brink: "For I am sure that neither death, nor life, . . . nor things present, nor things to come, . . . nor anything else in all creation, will be able to separate us from the love of God in Christ Jesus our Lord" (Rom. 8:38-39).

At this point Jesus' parable of the leaven instructs us again. The love of God through Christ becomes the "good leaven." Because of this love nothing, even cancer, will be able to separate us from God. Yet this love does even more. As we respond in love to God we are also united with each other. Even as earthen vessels, cracked and damaged, our love as husband, wife, and children has vitality because it is fueled by God's love. Nothing in all creation, even cancer, can overcome it. Even when the bad leaven of cancer has done its worst, the good leaven of God's love sustains us, to the end.

Sexuality and Mortality ──────

My *beloved speaks and says to me:*
"Arise, my love, my fair one,
  and come away;
for lo, the winter is past,
  the rain is over and gone.
The flowers appear on the earth,
  the time of singing has come,
and the voice of the turtledove
  is heard in our land. . . .
Arise, my love, my fair one,
  and come away."

Song of Solomon 2:10-13

I HAVE CHOSEN THIS PASSAGE as the starting point
for my reflections on love and sexuality because it

describes very beautifully the feelings Ruth and I have had for each other across thirteen years, before cancer. Our relationship then was mostly "time[s] of singing." We built a life together as we completed our education and began our careers. But our physical relationship was also very important. We reveled in each other's presence and eagerly awaited our shared time together.

In the six years since my diagnosis, the nature of our relationship has changed — subtly at first, more noticeably at some times than at others. But overall the "time of singing" now seems long ago and far away. Understanding and expressing this change is difficult. I find help in another Old Testament passage, one of the most familiar stories in the Bible: the story of Adam and Eve.

> Then the LORD God said, "It is not good that the man should be alone; I will make him a helper fit for him. . . ." And the rib which the LORD God had taken from the man he made into a woman and brought her to the man. Then the man said,
>
> "This at last is bone of my bones
> and flesh of my flesh . . ."
>
> Therefore a man leaves his father and his mother and cleaves to his wife, and they become

one flesh. And the man and his wife were both
naked, and were not ashamed. (Gen. 2:18, 22-25)

The beginning of the story of Adam and Eve is
remarkably similar to the passage from the Song
of Solomon with which we began. Here the
author of Genesis describes the beginning of
Adam and Eve's "time of singing." But this harmonious time does not last long. In Genesis 3
Adam and Eve eat from "the fruit of the tree"
(vv. 3, 6). As a result of this rebellious act, they
are banished from the garden. God declares their
punishment: instead of happy and harmonious
life in the garden, pain in childbirth and hard
toil will now be Eve's and Adam's fates (vv. 15,
16, 19). The perfect union of "one flesh" is
broken.

The story of Adam and Eve's unity and fall
parallels in striking ways the changes that have
occurred in our relationship. We too have experienced the joy of oneness and intimacy in our
life together, the "time of singing" described here
and in the Song of Solomon. But the onset of
cancer has changed everything, including our
physical relationship. The joyful union of "one
flesh" is torn apart by disease. "Till death us do
part" reads the traditional wedding ritual; but

now cancer has parted us and stands constantly between us.

The changes are pervasive. Clearly, extended periods of treatment and hospitalization damage our physical relationship. It is difficult to imagine the joy of physical intimacy when I am hooked up to I.V. pumps or vomiting because of chemotherapy. But even when I am not undergoing treatment, my cancer still comes between us. The old sense of freedom and spontaneity is gone. The intravenous catheter in my chest and enlarged nodes across my body are all-too-evident reminders of my cancer. Ruth can't embrace me without feeling these signs of illness. My cancer has become a wedge which drives us apart against our wills.

We have lost the unity and wholeness of our "pre-cancer" relationship, the "time[s] of singing" that we used to enjoy. Enduring this broken oneness becomes as difficult as living with the cancer itself. Ruth's summary of the situation captures the way we often feel: "Get well or get out!" We yearn for the wholeness as a couple which we had before. Memories of the way things used to be, of physical intimacy free from the shadow of cancer, haunt us. We have lost the state of union in which we could be naked and not ashamed. Our garden of Eden and our "time of singing" seem far behind us now and impossible to recapture. And the future is bleak. When Adam and Eve's relationship was broken because of their disobedince, death was introduced into human experience: "You are dust, and to dust you shall return" (Gen. 3:19). For Ruth and me, the wedge now driven between us by cancer will eventually lead to the final separation (in this life, at least) of death.

When we reflect on the story of Adam and Eve, we usually focus on the Fall, humanity's separation from God through our own deliberate choice. I am mystified when I try to find a correlation between this aspect of the story and my own present life. Am I in some sense responsible for my cancer? Have I not thought enough positive thoughts to overcome the malignant cells? Did too much worrying in the past contribute to lowered immunity and weaken my ability to fight the disease in its early stages? I do not know, and I do not expect ever to know. The *origins* of my cancer are a mystery, but the *results* of it are clear enough. And these results, at least, parallel those of the Fall as described in Genesis. My cancer has damaged our married life and our physical relationship, and it has radically introduced us to death.

The story of Adam and Eve is helpful in understanding the destructiveness of cancer in our married life, but it offers very little hope. Adam and Eve never returned to Eden; their "time of singing" had passed. But we may find some hope in a later passage from the Song of Solomon:

> Set me as a seal upon your heart,
> as a seal upon your arm;
> for love is strong as death . . .
>
> (8:6)

Is there a clue here that can help us beyond the Fall, beyond the separation caused by chronic illness? As with Adam and Eve, death and pain will not disappear from our life as a couple. Yet Jesus' incarnation points to a new dimension: God comes to be with us in our pain. We do not have to unravel all the mysteries of the Fall to appreciate that Christ is with us in my illness. St. Paul writes, "For if many died through one man's [Adam's] trespass, much more have the grace of God and the free gift in the grace of that one man Jesus Christ abounded for many" (Rom. 5:15). For Paul, Christ is the new Adam who overcomes sin and death. We can even rejoice in our suffering, because "suffering produces endurance," which produces character, which produces hope, "and hope does not disappoint us, because God's love has been poured into our hearts through the Holy Spirit which has been given to us" (5:3-5).

Thus suffering eventually leads to hope, if we accept God's gift of love. What meaning does this have for Ruth and me as we struggle with the destructive effects of cancer in our relationship? First, God's love does not necessarily end all suffering and pain; it does not even necessarily postpone death. Jesus himself suffered and died. The incarnation was cloaked in pain but led to victory over pain and death. For now we must learn to live with the pain, both my physical pain and the pain of our broken relationship. But we also need to recognize that the pain and feeling of separation are not the end. Our time of singing may be over for now, but God's last act has not yet been completed.

Second, we can seek to live our remaining life together under the reflection of the new Eden. This is an ambivalent existence: we continue to live in this world where death is a reality, but we also believe that resurrection stands beyond. We stand between the times, regretting our losses but cultivating our hopes.

This life between the times is terribly difficult. Sometimes between treatments, when I am feeling well, we can momentarily almost forget my cancer. Ruth and I can enjoy each other again, and our old wholeness — our "time of singing" — begins to return. But then the singing fades. I contract pneumonia following chemotherapy and am hospitalized for twelve days. The doctors are unable to determine the cause of a high fever. I become once again a patient, not a lover. The wedge is driven between us again, and each time Ruth wonders whether I will recover.

Gradually, though, we have come to accept the physical limitations. Through God's grace we have decided that it is better to be together — even without wholeness — than to be separated. We have come to this awareness only after grieving for the time of singing we have lost. But now we can celebrate what we still have together. Loving through the pain is possible, through grace.

Needing Friends and Being a Friend ———————

IN RECENT YEARS, since cancer struck, I have become more aware of the role of friendship in living. Much of my life I have been a loner, neither depending upon nor getting close to others. Perhaps the roots of this pattern stretch back to my moving every three years or so as I was growing up. With the advent of chemotherapy, however, I have gained new appreciation for friendship and its role in human living. Paul's description of the body as one, with many members (1 Cor. 12:12), has found new significance in my life.

One result of my encounter with cancer has been an increased awareness of my need for other people. Others who wrestle with illness have similar experiences. I recall overhearing a conversation in a clinic waiting room. A young pharmacist from a small town in Arkansas was recounting how his colleagues had pitched in, allowing him to keep his pharmacy open while he received treatment for cancer. He was amazed at their generosity as well as grateful for their help.

Like this pharmacist, I have found that I do not stand alone. Even when healthy, I am only one member of Christ's body; when ill, my dependence on others becomes inescapable. Numerous tasks which I did for myself before, I now need help in doing. Raking leaves and washing the car are more difficult than in the past, even on "good days." Most problematic have been childcare arrangements and transportation to tests or treatment away from home. We have necessarily called on friends and family for help. Previously we would have felt we were "imposing." Now we have no choice. The children need to attend school and maintain their own schedules as much as possible. And people have been ready to assist us when asked. We have tried very hard not to ask more than necessary, but often people seem glad to be called on for help. Driving me to the hospital, running to the store, or babysitting become concrete expressions of caring — opportunities to experience the reality that we are all members of Christ's one body and that we all need the support of others.

Though we rarely think about it, Jesus also needed friends. For me the most poignant illustration of this need came on the night of his arrest. As he went to the garden to pray, he asked Peter, James, and John to watch with him (Mark 14:33-34). Jesus asked for help from his disciples! He needed them. They fell asleep and let him down, but Jesus returned to them three times. Throughout his active ministry, the disciples were his almost constant companions. How painful then this failure by those closest to him must have been. Even while he was on the cross, Jesus continued to be concerned about friends and family, telling the beloved disciple to care for his mother Mary (John 19:26-27). To the end of his physical life, Jesus knew and attended to human relationships.

Friendship is underscored elsewhere in the Bible as well. It is essential to Paul in his ministry. To the Philippians he declares, "I thank my God in all my remembrance of you, . . . thankful for your partnership in the gospel from the first day until now" (1:3, 5). In the same letter Paul writes of Timothy's support: "But Timothy's worth you know, how as a son with a father he has served with me in the gospel" (2:22). Surely Paul's own life reflected his theology of many members but one body.

My struggle with cancer has provided differing experiences with friends. Some old friends, perhaps threatened by their own mortality, have pulled away. Others, however, have sought to rekindle old relationships, drawing upon past foundations but responding now to the new dimension of cancer. The body of Christ cannot become static. It must grow and change, or wither and die. I have sensed the pain as some of these friends have shared their tears with me and grappled with their own finitude. This reforging of old bonds can be difficult and painful, but it has provided me with a much-needed link to my past before cancer and with a bridge to the future. I believe the rekindling has also brought growth and new insights to those who have struggled with me. We have grown together, as Christ's body.

Beyond restructuring old relationships, my life with cancer has also brought me into contact with new friends, many of whom have already had encounters with this disease. Recreation therapy volunteers in oncology wards give their time, talents, and support freely. What better place to hear a harpsichord concert of Christmas music one week before Christmas day? Touched by cancer themselves, many of these individuals understand the struggles Ruth and I go through. Nurses and staff in short-stay centers and on cancer floors have also been very supportive. Often they have become a nurturing family away from home, who remember your last visit and the funny story you told last time. Church members have reached out too, some from their own reservoirs of pain, with prayers, food, childcare, money. And sometimes the tender word or deed comes from the one least expected. In all these cases we experience one of the miracles of the body of Christ. Unlike our physical bodies, it can add new members as it develops. Thus all can be enriched.

Waiting: Waste vs. Preparation

ANYONE WHO UNDERGOES long-term therapy for chronic illness learns to wait. You may not like it, but waiting is as much a part of your experience as tests and treatment. Ruth and I have sometimes joked about the need to hurry up and wait. After a while one pays little attention to the scheduled appointment time. The only question becomes, How long will the wait be? Fifteen minutes or four hours? As the doctor's secretary once told me, "It doesn't matter what time you're scheduled for. Come prepared to spend the day." So I go equipped to wait, taking books to read, bills to pay, cards to write.

Waiting becomes perpetual. Perhaps our society's emphasis upon "doing something" exacerbates our situation. We need to be active to maintain our identity as doers. We perceive waiting to be valueless. When we are inactive, we believe we are wasting our time, not being productive. We feel worthless.

What happens to us when we are continually confronted with such forced waiting? Usually frustration and anger mount. We have other appointments to keep, other plans. The longer we wait, the more frustrated we become. Having to receive chemotherapy or other treatment is bad enough. Prolonged waiting adds insult to injury. Our patience wears thin, and we lose sight of the goal of our treatment. We can understand the impatience of the people of Israel, when Moses tarried for forty days on the mountain. Fed up with waiting, they said to Aaron: "Come, make us gods who will go before us. As for this fellow Moses who brought us up out of Egypt, we don't know what has happened to him" (Exod. 32:1, NIV). In our impatience we too may turn away from God. When God's pace seems too slow, we may seek faith healers or other doctors. We may vent our rage against God. We may lose hope, give up. And often we lash out at those around us, even our family and supportive friends.

Our impatience can thus be destructive. But

it can also carry positive possibilities. As long as we are impatient we still have life and energy. All hope is not lost. In John's account of the man by the pool of Bethesda (John 5:2-16), the man is perhaps too patient. He has waited for thirty-eight years to get into the curing waters but has never gotten there quickly enough. Jesus short-circuits the process, declaring simply, "Rise, take up your pallet, and walk" (5:8). Sometimes we too need to become impatient with the waiting and to take charge. But we need to learn self-control, to know when to be patient and when to be impatient. This ability can help us to manage waiting constructively. It brings us some measure of control. Once, while waiting for chemotherapy on Labor Day weekend, I was told that my chart couldn't be located. Two hours later it was still missing. Had I not continued to press for action, I could have waited all day. Finally arrangements were made to use the copy of the doctor's orders kept in the pharmacy. My chart was not found until the following day. (As the hand-lettered sign I kept on my desk during graduate school reads, "Victory is a question of stamina!") Too often, though, I suspect I have been too patient, not pressing for action when it would have been appropriate to do so.

A woman whose husband was hospitalized for complications from lymphoma shared this story with me. Her husband, who was experiencing great pain, needed a transfusion. The young resident on duty that night was hesitant to use the patient's catheter tube for the transfusion, wanting instead to insert an I.V. needle. He wavered back and forth, unable to make up his mind. Finally the wife said to him, "You have three choices: start the transfusion using the catheter yourself, call someone who will, or forget the transfusion." Someone was eventually found who would connect the catheter tube. That night, the wife said, she determined never to wait helplessly again. She had learned to manage waiting, to regain self-control.

For me, another outcome of waiting has been a new appreciation for the significance of prayer and meditation. Jesus' prayer in the Garden of Gethsemane stands as a model for us here. Waiting for his own arrest, he prayed to his Father. Jesus was honest with God. Mark declares that he was "greatly distressed and troubled" and then records Jesus' own words: "My soul is very sorrowful, even to death" (14:33-34). Like us, Jesus was troubled as he faced suffering, but unlike us he readily expressed his feelings in prayer to

God. He knew the value of prayer and meditation. In the garden he used his time of waiting to gain strength for events to come.

These reflections indicate that our waiting can become a time of preparation, even though we may not know exactly what we are preparing for. Waiting need not be merely wasted time, a period of "just floating" when our lives are on hold. We are not obliged to become just prisoners whose lives are out of control. In the Exodus story, we find the Hebrew people's entry into the Promised Land delayed for forty years. True, the delay is because of their own faithlessness. But the forty-year wait becomes a period of preparation for the tasks of settlement facing them. The time of waiting thus becomes bridge time, linking the past with the future.

For us, too, waiting need not be equated with waste. In our waiting we can learn patience and controlled assertiveness. Prayer and meditation come to have renewed significance. And waiting beomes preparation for whatever lies ahead.

Disability: Wilderness
Experience and Temptation ─────

"WORK, FOR THE NIGHT IS COMING, Work thro'
the morning hours; . . . Work, for the night is
coming, When man's work is done."* In our
society our work or job is important to us. In
many ways, we are what we do. One of the first
things I ask when I meet someone new is "What
do you do?" For most of us, our jobs mold our
identities. Our "forty hours" each week shape
who we are at home or church, with friends, on
vacation.

But what happens to us when we are unable
to work, when we are disabled? The transition
from able to disabled is usually difficult. Our

---

* *Cokesbury Worship Hymnal*, no. 201.

perceptions of ourselves suffer when we are not able to do our usual work. When I am asked about my teaching, I have to explain that I am on disability leave — the words always seem strange to me. I am taking a sabbatical not of my own choosing! Life seems "on hold"; the pause or stop button has been pushed.

Reflection upon the Gospels may help us to find meaning in this state of disability or limbo. Labor is recognized as worthwhile in the Bible: "The laborer deserves his wages," Jesus said (Luke 10:7). But we should also recognize that, to our knowledge, Jesus himself never held a steady job as a mature adult. He taught, healed, and traveled, but he was not an official priest. His ministry was never for pay. While Jesus stayed busy, he also periodically withdrew for meditation and renewal. In one period of withdrawal — his temptation before the beginning of his active ministry — we find clues which can assist us in our periods of disability. Our periods of extended illness and disability can be like Jesus' withdrawal into the wilderness, and temptation can be present for us as well. Christ's experience can illuminate our own.

Matthew reports that when Christ went into the wilderness, he "was led up by the Spirit"

(4:1). The Spirit leads Jesus into temptation. I find this difficult to comprehend. Yet Jesus' experience in the wasteland clarifies his mission and becomes the launching pad for his ministry. Might illness and disability also prepare us for something, whether for continued life or for death? Is there some leading of the Spirit here which we need to comprehend?

Both Matthew and Luke record the devil's challenge to turn stone into bread as the first temptation of Jesus (Matt. 4:3; Luke 4:3). If he alleviated physical hunger, surely Jesus would attract a large following. Yet Jesus replies, "It is written, 'Man shall not live by bread alone, but by every word that proceeds from the mouth of God'" (Matt. 4:4). Jesus won't ignore physical needs, of course, but deeper needs will direct his ministry.

In times of illness and disability, we are preoccupied with our physical needs. Our pain and suffering are great, and we come to think of hardly anything else. I have discovered that my illness at times almost overwhelms Ruth and me. We lose touch with friends, with our children, with each other — even with ourselves. Illness swallows up everything else. We concentrate on appointments, treatments, tests. We eat and sleep cancer. All of this is understandable, yet Jesus' reply presses us beyond our physical pain. Even physical healing itself would not solve all our problems. Jesus is indeed concerned about my physical pain, but he presses me beyond it to something more — the word of God.

In his second temptation (following Matthew's order), Jesus is challenged by the devil to throw himself down from the pinnacle of the Temple (Matt. 4:5-6). The temptation of miracles! How familiar this one is to those of us who are ill or disabled. Like the children of Israel, who murmured against Moses when they lacked water in the wilderness, we "put the LORD to the proof" (see Exod. 17:1-7). We cry out for miraculous healing.

I recall a young woman in one of Ruth's early parishes who almost bled to death after childbirth. Across several tense days her family and church prayed for healing. Her husband and their three children under the age of five needed her. After a fast late-night transfer to a major medical center, surgeons operated and saved her life. Soon she was back home again. But not in church. Strangely she and her family rarely attended. The miracle came; the deeper faith did not.

I do not want to be misunderstood here. I

too want to be healed. Yet Jesus points out a deeper truth that emphasis upon miracles alone may obscure. We must focus first upon God and not upon miracles.

Jesus' third temptation involves power over "all the kingdoms of the world" (Matt. 4:8-10). Political power is the attraction here. How can this speak to me in my illness? I don't seek political power. But I would like power over my illness. Consider the millions of dollars and countless hours spent each year on cancer research. Money and time well spent, I believe. Yet even the quest to discover cures for cancer can mislead us. Do we not shower adulation upon our medical heroes? No matter how great their success, they must not replace God. All of us will eventually die, whether of cancer, accident, or "old age." And whatever our age or condition, we are called to worship only God.

Illness and disability may thus be a time when we face our own temptations. Our withdrawal may enable us to grow in our faith as we wrestle with our disability. Without minimizing our yearning for an end to physical pain, for miraculous healing and power over our illness, the Gospel accounts of Jesus' temptation point us beyond the physical to God our maker.

Difficult Decisions

THE PAIN OF CHRONIC ILLNESS is not all physical. Time and again one must make decisions about which treatments (if any) to try, which doctors to consult, which medical center to choose. The consent forms and background data on alternative treatments become a regular part of life. Mental fatigue and confusion confront us, as well as illness itself.

How then do we decide? In the Gospels Jesus presents two parables which are instructive. In the first, a rich man with abundant crops has nowhere to store them, for his barns are overflowing. What will he do? "I will pull down my barns, and build larger ones; and there I will store all my grain and my goods." But note also the following verse: "And I will say to my soul, Soul, you have ample goods laid up for many years; take your ease, eat, drink, be merry." Yet that very night, Jesus continues, the man dies (Luke 12:16-21).

In the parable Jesus is addressing the danger of covetousness. Given this focus, the message may not seem to relate to my decision making about medical treatment. What is significant for our context is the final verse: "So is he who lays up treasure for himself, and is not rich toward God." The foundation for decision making, this verse suggests to me, becomes our relationship with God. The basic mistake of the rich fool is that his priorities are reversed. He trusts in himself and his abilities to provide for his own welfare. Before one decides about new barns or new treatment, then, one needs to clarify one's priorities. The rich fool's problem was not difficulty in decision making; it was that his decisions were grounded in himself, not in God.

The one-talent man in another parable of Jesus (Matt. 25:14-30) faces a different problem. Whereas the rich fool easily makes his decision to tear down his barns and rebuild, the man who receives one talent (more than a laborer would earn in fifteen years) is paralyzed by anxiety. He is afraid and opts to hide what he has received rather than risk it through investing. Where the rich fool is too self-confident in decision making, the one-talent man is too insecure. Because of his fear of failure, he is not the good steward his master expects.

In my own decision making, I seem to combine the worst characteristics of the rich fool and the one-talent man. When each new treatment plan is presented, I seek out the facts. I gather data, reams of it. My brother, a physician, supplies me with relevant medical journal articles and "translations" of the technical jargon, as needed. My filing cabinets, if not my barns, overflow. Soon I become a well-educated medical "consumer." I have the facts so *I* can decide. But still I am confused. I rarely feel that I have enough data or the right facts. At least once I have had directly contradictory courses of treatment suggested by different oncologists. What do I do then? I feel like the one-talent man. I am afraid to decide. I don't trust my own judgment. My anxiety mounts. Should I seek still another opinion? Whom do I trust?

I find the key to my dilemma in this last sentence: Whom do I trust? I am driven beyond the immediate decision itself to the issue of relationships. As Jesus teaches in his parable of the rich fool, basic issues of trust and priorities under-lie our decisions. For me, the basic question is, Which doctor has earned my trust in the past? My decision about future treatment thus hinges upon what has gone before. For example, on one occasion I had to decide whether or not to follow a doctor's suggestion that we repeat treatment with Fludarabine Phosphate, an experimental drug. Although this drug had initially brought good results, it had then led to complications from which I almost died. I asked another oncologist for a second opinion. This doctor had first placed me upon Fludarabine Phosphate and then stopped it in favor of conventional chemotherapy. He responded with a solid "No!" to further treatment with that drug. Because I had grown to trust this doctor, I chose to follow his advice. Beyond the medical data stood the person.

Trusting one's physician thus can help in the process of decision making. But even this will not resolve all problems. The doctor one trusts will sometimes be uncertain which treatment to pursue. And, as my trusted physician has emphasized to me, even the best oncologist has limited medical tools. No cure is known for my kind of lymphoma. My doctor is thus recommending treatment options which may help me to live better, longer. But he does not promise a cure.

Within this context, then, I continually must decide. Which treatment next (if any)? For how long? Here I am led again to the teaching of Jesus. In Luke's Gospel, immediately following the parable of the rich fool, Jesus tells his disciples: "Do not be anxious about your life, what you shall eat, nor about your body, what you shall put on. For life is more than food, and the body more than clothing" (12:22-23). Anxiety itself does not help us. "And which of you by being anxious can add a cubit to his span of life? If then you are not able to do as small a thing as that, why are you anxious about the rest?" (vv. 25-26). My anxiety over choosing treatments may be natural, but in itself it may not be helpful. Sometimes anxiety can paralyze, as in the case of the one-talent man.

Still, the anxiety does underscore that the stakes are high. The servant wrestling over what to do with his talent knew this too. In a positive way, the anxiety may press me beyond the immediate decision to the question, Whom do I finally trust? Do I trust myself and my judgment, as the rich fool did? Do I feel paralyzed, unwilling to act, like the one-talent man? Can I place my ultimate fate in the hands of even my best doctors? With the hearers of Jesus' parable about the rich fool, I am driven back to my foundation. Finally I must ask myself: Am I "rich toward God"? Do I trust the God who provides for the ravens and the lilies of the field also to provide food and clothing for me? Even more, do I trust this God to sustain me, even with my cancer? Too often I am among the "men of little faith" (Luke 12:28). But I have at least glimpsed what faith involves. It can buoy me up as I decide about my treatment and help me to recognize that my life is not finally in my own — or my doctors' — hands. Through surrendering to God, in faith, I can move beyond anxiety to fulfilled living, for whatever period of time. I can move beyond the pain of decision making.

As I observed earlier, this theology of surrender brings new-found freedom. Trust in God liberates me from the anxiety associated with choosing. The words of the gospel hymn say it best:

> Be not dismayed whate'er betide, God will
> take care of you;
> beneath his wings of love abide, God will
> take care of you.

No matter what may be the test, God will
	take care of you;
lean, weary one, upon his breast, God will
	take care of you.

God will take care of you, through every day,
	o'er all the way;
he will take care of you, God will
	take care of you.*

* "God Will Take Care of You," *United Methodist Hymnal*
(1989), no. 130.

Material Things
and the Natural World —————

ONE INTRIGUING ASPECT of my experience with cancer has been my attitude toward the natural world and toward material things. While one dimension of my living with cancer has pressed me into spiritual reflection, another has led me to a new appreciation of the natural and the material. During stays in the hospital, I have enjoyed doing sand art and painting figurines — activities I would never have participated in before. At home, washing the car, raking leaves, and doing odd jobs bring a sense of accomplishment, even enjoyment. And walks through the state forest or a boat ride through the morning fog have brought me a sense of melancholy, but also peace.

What about this attraction to the material and natural world? Sometimes I have considered it a welcome distraction, though perhaps a denial of my cancer. When I work on my son's bicycle or winterize my outboard motor, I can temporarily forget my illness as I wrestle with steel wrenches, rubber tires, and gear oil. Here is something elemental and basic, where I don't have to ponder the meaning of living and dying. Do the job right and that bicycle and old outboard will run almost forever. As I concentrate on nuts and bolts, the hospital room with ticking I.V. pumps seems far away. I can escape for a while.

Even in the images which have become important to me during my illness, escape through the natural and material world emerges powerfully. Using visualization techniques presented by Bernie S. Siegel, M.D., in *Love, Medicine and Miracles*,* I see myself resting beneath a waterfall as the pure cascading water streams across my body. I feel the clear water washing away my cancer. Images of escape are also explicit in the poem "Home" which I wrote several winters ago:

* Bernie S. Siegel, M.D., *Love, Medicine and Miracles* (Harper & Row, 1986).

My boat rocks, shivers on the open lake
before the dawn.
Alone in black.
Until it's chased by prying finger light,
itself still gray.
I need not move to watch the wispy beams
capture rising mist from off my bow.
When far from shore dawn draws its breath,
I'm home.

A paradox has arisen for me. As my poem illustrates, my return to nature does suggest escape. But through my experience with nature, I am drawn beyond it into the spiritual realm. Such poetic reflections and experiences have brought me renewal from the exhaustion of dealing with my disease. Hope is present here as the pure water splashes across my shoulders. And "when far from shore dawn draws its breath," I find hope and peace — wherever home is.

Usually we don't think much about Jesus' relation with physical things or the natural world. We may imagine his playing in the fields or working with wood in his father's shop when he was a child, but when he became a man he put aside such things. Or did he? Throughout the Gospels Jesus draws again and again from the natural world to illustrate his teaching: the tree will be known by its fruit; the sower casts seeds; "I send you out as lambs in the midst of wolves" — to mention just a few examples (Luke 6:43-44; 8:4-8; 10:3).

Physical objects also play an important role in Jesus' ministry and teaching. A patch from unshrunk cloth will rip away if sewn onto an old garment. Five loaves and two fish are used to feed five thousand. A lost coin causes a frantic search until it is found (Matt. 9:16; Luke 9:13-17; 15:8-9).

Jesus, then, emerges as an acute observer of the natural world and the physical things around him, and ordinary physical objects play an important role throughout his life and ministry. His ministry begins following his temptation in the wilderness, where, among other things, Satan challenges him to turn a stone to bread (Luke 4:3). In John's Gospel his first miracle involves turning water into wine at the wedding feast in Cana of Galilee (2:1-11). And near the end of his ministry, he uses two everyday items to create a service we still celebrate as the center of our faith:

> Now as they were eating, Jesus took bread, and blessed, and broke it, and gave it to the

disciples and said, "Take, eat; this is my body."
And he took a cup, and when he had given thanks
he gave it to them, saying, "Drink of it, all of you;
for this is my blood of the covenant, which is
poured out for many for the forgiveness of sins."
(Matt. 26:26-28)

Reflecting upon Jesus' own life and ministry,
I am discovering that my encounters with the
material and natural world may not be so far
removed from my spiritual quest after all. Tools,
tires, and foggy lakes are parts of God's world.
Sometimes they become a way for me to escape
from my illness for a while, but sometimes they
also lead me toward spiritual renewal. The
Psalmist knew well how the natural and material
could connect us to spiritual refreshment:

The LORD is my shepherd, I shall not want;
    he makes me lie down in green pastures.
He leads me beside still waters;
    he restores my soul.
He leads me in paths of righteousness
    for his name's sake.

Even though I walk through the valley of the
    shadow of death,

I fear no evil;
for thou art with me;
    thy rod and thy staff,
    they comfort me.

Thou preparest a table before me
    in the presence of my enemies;
thou anointest my head with oil,
    my cup overflows.
Surely goodness and mercy shall follow me
    all the days of my life;
and I shall dwell in the house of the Lord
    for ever.

(Psalm 23)

Sick Humor

KNOWING THAT I WOULD UNDERSTAND, a pastor friend shared a story with me about a recent hospital visit. When she arrived, the patient was out of his room, so she decided to leave a note. Looking for notepaper in her purse, she could find only a pad imprinted with the words: "Notepad, notepad, on my desk, guess whose life is the biggest mess!" Not sure that he would appreciate that message, she tore it off the paper and jotted a brief "hello." Later she visited again and related the story. "You should have left it," he said. "I love it!"

A Lutheran pastor told me about the hospital stay of a parishioner. Following surgery and several hours in surgical intensive care, the man was wheeled to his room. There he discovered an arrangement of flowers sent by colleagues. When the patient saw the flowers, he laughed so hard that, as he said later, he almost pulled out his stitches. In the pot was an assortment of dead mums, all sprayed black. The man's friends knew him well. Their touch of humor brightened his days of recuperation.

Our family has laughingly created our own takeoff on an anti-drug commercial on television. In the ad the narrator holds up an egg and declares "This is your brain." Next we see a heated frying pan and hear, "This is drugs." Finally, as he cracks the egg into the sizzling grease, the spokesperson intones, "This is your brain on drugs!" We had discussed this commercial with our two sons. Then one day after chemotherapy, when I was having trouble remembering what happened the day before, Ruth said, "This is your brain on drugs!" We all laughed, despite the situation.

"Sick humor." Often visitors to someone who is seriously ill wonder about the appropriateness of a joke or funny story. In normal life they would readily share it with the one who is ill, but, after all, illness is serious business. Being hospitalized or confined at home is no laughing matter. Or is it? The underlying question is the appropriateness of humor among those who are ill. The visitor doesn't want to make the "patient" uncomfortable or uneasy, so visits often assume a somber tone. This concern for the patient's welfare is commendable, but it can sometimes be misguided, as the opening stories suggest. The key lies in knowing the patient and the present circumstances. Being sensitive to the patient's needs is essential.

Sometimes humor arises from the absurdity of the situation, as in the story of Abraham, the "father" of the Israelites. When he was told that Sarah his wife would bear a son, he "fell on his face and laughed." After all Abraham himself was an old man (one hundred) and Sarah was ninety. Surely this was a bad joke! But God persisted (Gen. 17:15-19). The following chapter relates a slightly different account of the story. In this account Sarah overheard Abraham's conversation with the Lord (or God's three messengers), and *she* "laughed to herself." But the Lord was listening and asked Abraham, "Why did Sarah laugh . . . ? Is anything too hard for the LORD?" (18:1-14).

Was Abraham's and Sarah's laughter appropriate? The text does not directly address God's response to Abraham. But it does explore the laughing of Sarah. According to Genesis, Sarah denied laughing at God's announcement, "for she was afraid" (18:15). The surprise word that she will become pregnant yields laughter, but then fear and denial follow. Was the laughter appropriate? Did she offend God? The text leaves us wondering about God's reaction, yet it is clear that Sarah communicates with God through her laughter and that God responds. God accepts Sarah — laughter, fear, and all — then proceeds with the divine plan; she will bear a son and "be a mother of nations" (17:16). Yet the most telling clue to God's response is found in the name which God gives the child: "You shall call his name Isaac" (17:19). In Hebrew "Isaac" means "he laughs." Frederick Buechner, in his book *Telling the Truth*, captures the essence of this divine reaction to Abraham and Sarah:

> So you can say that God not only tolerated their laughter but blessed it and in a sense joined in it himself, which makes it a very special laughter indeed.*

May there be a hint here for us, that through our laughter — even unwittingly — we also can

* Frederick Buechner, *Telling the Truth* (Harper & Row, 1977), p. 53.

communicate with God? Our laughter reaches out beyond our fear and pain. It may indeed be appropriate, opening us to God's will.

This story about Sarah also alerts us to the role of surprise in laughter. Sometimes we who are ill become prisoners of our self-pity and boredom. We need something to break us out. Once after chemotherapy Ruth and the boys playfully told me, "You look terrible!" Then we laughed. Another family joke has grown from the discussion of my life insurance policies. When Ruth mentioned to Eric that fortunately I had purchased a good amount of insurance years ago, Eric replied, "Let's waste him!" Again we laughed. The surprise comment brought comic relief to the situation. I also remember being hospitalized shortly before Halloween. When I walked into the hall that morning, I was surprised to see the walls decorated and most of the nurses and doctors dressed as ghosts or goblins. The surprise brought a smile and a sense of release. Humor can become the best medicine, if it opens us to new insights, strength, and hope. Laughter can be the trigger for new healing, whether spiritual, psychological, or physical.

Humor may also restore a sense of control to those who are ill. At a time when we feel most powerless, if we can laugh at our disease, or our treatment or our appearance, then we in some measure control it. We are not completely victims. Through laughing we can rise above our suffering. As Ruth commented, "If you lose your sense of humor, you're lost." We often hear people say "I laughed so hard I cried!" But the opposite may be even more relevant for the seriously ill: "I cried so hard I laughed." Laughter may become the *bridge* from tears to renewal and hope. It can empower us when we feel like pawns of disease and circumstance.

We who are chronically ill need to laugh. We need "sick humor" — we need to be able to laugh *about* our illness. In the Sermon on the Plain found in the Gospel of Luke (which parallels in part Matthew's Sermon on the Mount), Jesus proclaims, "Blessed are you that weep now, for you shall laugh" (Luke 6:21). Indeed, our present laughter may even mirror the promised laughter in God's kingdom. The laughter in the hospital room may provide that "foretaste of glory divine" which Fanny J. Crosby describes in her famous hymn "Blessed Assurance."* It may help us to form a bridge between the present

* *Cokesbury Worship Hymnal*, no. 64.

hardships and the future victory. Our present laughter — or "sick humor" — may even become for us an incarnation of God's love, if we are open to it.

On the Road:
Journeying vs. Arriving ─────────

IN READING THE BIBLICAL WITNESS, I am often struck by the significance of journeying in Scripture. Moses and the chosen people travel for forty years in the wilderness. Jesus moves about continually and makes one last, momentous journey to Jerusalem. Paul's journeys are even better known. Reflecting upon these accounts, however, we discover that often, literally or figuratively, the journeys are incomplete.

Consider Moses. He is constantly "on the road" in the biblical accounts — fleeing from Pharaoh to the wilderness, returning to lead his people out of bondage in Egypt, then spending forty years sojourning in the Sinai Peninsula, camping out and moving on. Against outside enemies, internal revolt, hunger and thirst, Moses prevails. He leads his people to the edge of the Promised Land. Then the Lord takes Moses up to the mountaintop. The land promised to Abraham, Isaac, and Jacob spreads in a sweeping vista before Moses' eyes. But then come these words from the Lord: "I have let you see it with your eyes, but you shall not go over there." And the author of Deuteronomy continues, "So Moses the servant of the LORD died there in the land of Moab, according to the word of the LORD" (34:4-5).

How unfair! This leader survived confrontations with Pharaoh, rebellion among his own people, and forty years of desert wanderings, only to die at the gates of the Promised Land according to God's will. (Although he was 120 years old, Moses' "eye was not dim, nor his natural force abated" [Deut. 34:7].) Is *seeing* the Promised Land reward enough?

Moses is not alone in failing to reach his destination. St. Paul would certainly be a "frequent flyer" by today's standards. In his letter to the church at Rome he describes his plans to visit the Christians there. First, though, he must take a collection for the poor to Jerusalem. Then he will visit Rome, but only briefly: "I hope to see you in passing as I go to Spain, and to be sped on my journey there by you, once I have enjoyed your company for a little" (Rom. 15:24). Probably Paul never reached his Spanish destination. Arrested in Jerusalem, he arrived in Rome as a prisoner. Execution, not another journey, awaited him.

Jesus never travels far by Paul's and Moses' standards. But he too is constantly on the move: "the Son of man has nowhere to lay his head" (Matt. 8:20). His last momentous journey is presented in detail by Luke. But Jesus' journeying days come to an end much sooner than either Moses' or Paul's, in Jerusalem where Paul will also be arrested.

Foreshortened journeys appear in the lives of all three men. In large measure their fulfillment comes through the events of the journey itself, not in arriving at a destination. Journeying is a life-style for these heroes of faith. Living is done while journeying, while they're on the road. Our society, by contrast, usually focuses upon arriving. We're a task-oriented culture which measures success by "having arrived." The process of getting there is often subsumed under the goal of arriving. If we don't arrive at the designated end of our journey, we fail. There are few rewards and reduced retirement benefits for those who don't complete the journey.

Living with chronic illness such as cancer, though, locates one outside our society's orientation. Often we will not have the opportunity to see and measure results of our labors. I have considered this point most when reflecting upon the growth of my two sons. Will I see them into adulthood? Probably not. But I am still journeying with them for a while. I have insights, opportunities, and challenges to share with them *because of* my illness. Can I make the most of these openings? Rather than celebrating their graduation into adulthood, I am seeking to celebrate each new day of development. Because I am on disability leave, I have more time, between treatments, to help them with school science projects and reports. And more time just to listen. Maybe *they* can learn something about patience, persistence, faith, and love through my illness. My younger son Nathan's regular prayers and my older son Eric's patient strength seem to indicate that they are growing.

For me, living has become a matter of journeying, not of arriving. Once while riding a bus to a doctor's appointment in Houston, a young man asked me where I was going. As the conversation continued, he learned that I had cancer, then blurted out, "Are you going to make it?" I replied, "The question is, how long?" None of us, of course, knows the answer to that question. Since I was diagnosed with cancer two healthy friends have died in car accidents. But with my cancer I in particular can't assume that I'll be healthy for the next twenty years and then have ten good years of retirement. I must seek fulfillment in the times between treatment and illness, the time now. I do have the opportunity to plant some seeds, though I must leave the outcome of the harvest to the Lord.

My experience has helped me to discover a dimension of faith I did not see before. Faith can learn to say, "It is finished," before we've reached what we thought and planned would be the end. Moses died on the mountaintop, seeing but not entering the Promised Land. Paul made it to Rome — as a prisoner — but not to Spain. Still, he (or one of his followers writing about him) could declare in 2 Timothy, "I have fought the good fight, I have finished the race, I have kept the faith" (4:7). And near the end of his earthly ministry, according to John's Gospel, Jesus said, "I glorified thee on earth, having accomplished the work which thou gavest me to do" (17:4).

Soon afterward, on the cross, he would cry out, "It is finished" (19:30).

Such faith means accepting closure before we've reached our projected goal. It means that Moses could trust Joshua, that Paul could trust Timothy, that Jesus could trust his disciples, and that I can trust my sons. The labors of the biblical heroes — and mine — have not been in vain. More than that, though, it means that they and I can trust the Lord of the harvest to carry on. God is faithful.

> Even though I walk through the valley of
>   the shadow of death,
>   I fear no evil;
> for thou art with me . . .
>
> (Psalm 23:4)

The God with whom we began our journey of faith will sustain us at its end and will continue the work in which we have labored. If we are faithful in our journey we need not worry about the destination.

Forgetting and
Remembering, Again ─────

RECENTLY I VISITED A FRIEND in the hospital as he was about to begin chemotherapy. Nine years ago he had undergone both surgery and chemotherapy for cancer. He had done very well until the past several months. Then a nagging cough and fatigue began to bother him. Tests confirmed that his cancer had recurred. During my visit he asked how I was doing. "Pretty well," I said. "No chemo now for seven months." Then he offered an insightful comment: "You fall back into denial, don't you?"

Could that be true? How, after six years of chemotherapy and surgery, could I still deny that I have cancer? But as I thought more about my friend's comment, I realized he was right. When things go well for a while, I do begin to forget. Like the Israelites in the desert who have experienced God's deliverance only a short time before, my memory of strength received from God and of the support of others begins to dim. I settle back into some semblance of normalcy. It's not just that I forget, but that I *want* to forget. I want to forget the pain of the treatments and the hours of tense waiting. The surgery and recovery. The weeks of pneumonia. But is forgetting really all that bad? Why not enjoy the present? "Sufficient unto the day is the evil thereof" (Matt. 6:34, KJV).

My forgetting is understandable and perhaps even somewhat therapeutic. But self-examination forces me to a deeper truth: forgetting also, I believe, involves my sin. Surely I should know the score, shouldn't take things for granted. But I tend to relapse. The hard-earned lessons of months past recede in memory. My prayer life and reflection on the Bible slip. My appreciation for the joys of the present diminishes. I find myself listening to the evening news playing on the television in the next room while our family eats supper together. I hear Nathan talking about his day at school and a girl in his class, but only after supper do I realize, through talking with

Ruth, that he had reported that he has a new girlfriend. Am I the same person who once said that the greatest legacy I could leave my sons was to be a good father to them now? Suddenly the evening news seems less important.

As I ponder my situation, different images of my spiritual life emerge. Is it like the tide, which ebbs and flows? Do I draw closer to God during crisis, only to recede as my condition improves for a time? Or is my spiritual life cyclical, moving from complacency to intense spiritual awareness and commitment, then back around to complacency again? Perhaps a better image is an ever-widening spiral, in which I move from spiritual insight to withdrawal and back around again, but hopefully at each cycle rising to a somewhat higher level, toward the eventual union with my Creator.

This image of the spiral is intriguing because it suggests to me that the dynamic of human existence continues as long as I live. With the founder of Methodism, John Wesley, I eye the goal of spiritual perfection. I also recall the words of Jesus: "You, therefore, must be perfect, as your heavenly Father is perfect" (Matt. 5:48). Still, the doubt and lack of understanding that was so frequently the disciples' experience returns. As I read the Gospels, I am amazed at how often they fail to understand. Even living daily with Jesus does not raise them to the plane of continual spiritual awareness. When they encounter a great storm on the Sea of Galilee, they fear for their lives and cry out to Jesus for help. "Why are you afraid, O men of little faith?" he queries when awakened from his nap in the boat (Matt. 8:23-26). Later, after teaching them a series of parables on the kingdom and giving detailed explanations of several parables (the parable of the sower and the parable of the farmer whose enemy sowed weeds in his field), Jesus asks his disciples, "Have you understood all this?" (13:51). The disciples' reply is simply "Yes." Yes, we understand. But shortly before Peter's famous confession of Jesus as the Christ, they stumble again. "O men of little faith, why do you discuss among yourselves the fact that you have no bread? Do you not yet perceive?" (16:8-9).

I find myself in the shoes of these twelve. I truly believe that I too have walked with Christ during my illness, yet I too so often falter. Nevertheless, I doubt that the answer lies in stressing spiritual perfection alone. John Wesley, in his early years, even sought to rate the intensity of his morning prayers, but he found no inner assurance through this practice. Instead, I am discovering that an emphasis upon surrender of my life to God provides a better focus. Then God's will becomes the key, rather than *my* striving for perfection. Perhaps a certain rhythm between intense spiritual awareness and return to the "normalcy" of everyday life is acceptable. Without doubt I recognize that my spiritual life will require lifelong nurture. I recall the words cut into stone beside the central arch at Rice University's Lovett Hall: "Love, beauty, joy and worship are forever building, unbuilding, and rebuilding in each man's soul." I would affirm this for my own faith, while praying that each rebuilding rises to a higher level than the last. Still, in the end, I trust not my own endeavor but God in Christ to bring me final peace.

Keeping Up the Fight
vs. Letting Go and Letting God ——

ACROSS THE YEARS friends and family members have urged me to keep on fighting. So far I have endured and even accepted countless scans, biopsies, and chemotherapy treatments. But so have others who have suffered much more than I have. Basically, I don't feel brave. I just do what I must, to get through. But why keep up this fight? I sometimes wonder. The prognosis isn't good. "Life" offers more of the same, or worse. As my wife and I have laughed — to keep from crying — maybe it doesn't get any better than this.

Ambiguity marks my reflections about my life. Does continued struggle reflect courageous faith in my Creator or a fearful clinging to the only life I know? During one hospital stay I shared a room with a critically ill man suffering with lung problems. "How old are you?" the nurse asked him. Gasping for breath, even on oxygen, he replied, "As old as I am going to get — sixty-three." But his daughter pleaded with him as she left for the night, "Don't give up, Daddy. You taught us to be fighters, and we are."

This overheard conversation has stuck with me. It illustrates the dilemma which many of us face. I live in part, I believe, because I love life. This realization has become clearer to me as my illness has progressed. I savor sunsets and time spent fishing with my sons. The smell of wood smoke recalls camping trips and laughter around the fire. Holding my wife still brings joy. Even with the pain and suffering, I still find much in life that is good. The simple things such as an evening walk through my neighborhood have taken on new significance. These experiences, I believe, rather than the fear of dying, keep me going.

Other dimensions of living also emerge. I live because I love my family. I want to see my sixteen- and eleven-year-old sons grow up. One of the most emotional moments for me since my diagnosis occurred on a trip home from the hospital. While my wife drove, I quietly sobbed, thinking that I might die before my older son Eric graduates from high school. Eric and Nathan need me, and this reality gives me motivation to live on. Love for my wife Ruth also motivates me. We have shared early lean years of schooling and launching careers. We've struggled with Ruth's pioneering work as a woman in parish ministry. Through it all, we've been there for each other. I don't want to leave Ruth now.

Still, the dilemma remains: How long should I struggle when days and hours for appreciating nature grow fewer, displaced by days and weeks of treatment? When time spent with family focuses more and more upon my illness and less and less upon activities we enjoy? Should I consent to twelve weeks of experimental therapy in Houston, Texas, which will separate me from my family and cause hardship for them, with uncertain results? St. Paul was able to write to his younger colleague Timothy: "For I am already on the point of being sacrificed; the time of my departure has come. I have fought the good fight, I have finished the race, I have kept the faith" (2 Tim. 4:6-7). Yet Paul's words underscore my question: Has the time of my departure come?

These words spoken by Jesus also echo in my mind: "Watch therefore, for you know neither the day nor the hour" (Matt. 25:13).

Through my illness and my reflections, the concept of "living enroute" has developed. Much of Jesus' own life was spent "on the road," in journeys around Galilee and in his last journey to Jerusalem. Indeed, in Luke this journey to Jerusalem occupies most of the Gospel and is the occasion for much of Jesus' teaching to his disciples. This "journey theology" has new significance for me these days. I still do not know, in the abstract, how long I should struggle or when to let go. Living becomes a daily challenge, with the future still unknown. I am sustained through my faith that Jesus has gone before, and that he will be present with me as I decide about future treatment or non-treatment. More and more I am learning to trust and serve him along the way.

Burial Plots: Rockpiles and Resurrection

"Why do you want to be planted in this rock-pile?" Mr. Russ asked me when we met. He is chief trustee for a little community cemetery near the Peaks of Otter, Virginia. Ruth and I tried to explain how the Peaks area had special significance for us. I camped there when growing up, and two sisters were married there. Maybe he understood. He and his wife Mary rode with us to see the cemetery. There we selected a beautiful plot on a hillside overlooking the Peaks. "Ashes to ashes, dust to dust," the old funeral ritual says. Even on the lush hillside these words raced through my mind.

For Ruth and me, a burial spot is important, yet not ultimate. In seeking a site we have looked for one reflecting who we are. To us a mountain-side is more peaceful than a well-manicured sub-urban plot. It reminds us of backpacking and camping with our sons, trips across many years. Here we feel closer to God. Of course, one is confronted with trade-offs in such decision making. Even in death our society seeks per-manence, with granite markers, perpetual care contracts, and moisture-proof caskets. Here on the hillside, though, the guarantees are less iron-clad. "What arrangements have been made to take care of the cemetery when you are gone?" Ruth asks. "No guarantees," Mr. Russ replies. "I'm trying to establish a fund for perpetual care, but no guarantees." He continues to talk about the old practice of using wood headstones and about cemeteries in the woods that are now over-grown.

Standing on the hillside, we look over the markers. Family plots, mostly. There are even some Harpers here, we discover. No relatives to our knowledge, but former owners of the adja-cent farm. One stone records a wedding date, then adds the words "Together in death." This phrase reminds me of the words of the biblical Ruth to Naomi, her mother-in-law: "Where you die I will die, and there will I be buried" (Ruth

1:17). Family plots were important in the Old Testament. Abraham bought the cave of Machpelah at Hebron in which to bury his wife Sarah (Gen. 23). Later he too was buried there, followed by his son Isaac and Isaac's wife Rebekah, and, later still, by his grandson Jacob and Jacob's wife Leah (49:31; 50:13). Abraham's family was "together in death."

As I recall our experiences at the Peaks Community Cemetery, I am reminded that death and burial are important themes for us as Christians, even before life's physical end. St. Paul uses them as symbols in his discussion of baptism. In Romans he declares:

> Do you not know that all of us who have been baptized into Christ Jesus were baptized into his death? We were buried therefore with him by baptism into death, so that as Christ was raised from the dead by the glory of the Father, we too might walk in newness of life. (6:3-4)

Our preliminary death is in our baptism, but how often do we understand baptism in this way? Perhaps more emphasis upon Paul's "baptism theology" would better prepare us for our physical death and reassure us of our reunion with Christ!

Events surrounding Christ's own death are also instructive for us. His preparations did not include elaborate planning for a tomb and for perpetual care. Rather, he focused upon preparing his disciples for his crucifixion and for their own continuing ministry.

> If any man would come after me, let him deny himself and take up his cross daily and follow me. For whoever would save his life will lose it; and whoever loses his life for my sake, he will save it. (Luke 9:23-24)

His own burial was hastily arranged, and he was laid to rest in a borrowed tomb by a distant admirer, Joseph of Arimathea (Mark 15:42-46). Don't we often reverse the order of Jesus' own concerns? We worry and plan about our own cemetery plots and perpetual care while giving too little attention to discipleship. Might Christ even be challenging us to use the period before our own death to prepare others to follow him?

Still, our emphasis upon plots does underscore our mortality. It underscores the fact that, despite our efforts and our wealth, we cannot save ourselves. Whether in an air-conditioned mausoleum or in a forgotten overgrown wayside

[97]

cemetery, our physical remains eventually decay. But here the experiences of Jesus and the emphasis of Paul instruct us again: for those who believe, the tomb — whether dug in sand or gold encased — is not the final resting place. As the young man in white told the women who had come to the tomb to anoint Jesus' body, "He has risen, he is not here" (Mark 16:6). As Jesus told his disciples in John's Gospel, "And when I go and prepare a place for you, I will come again and will take you to myself, that where I am you may be also" (John 14:3).

As Christians, then, our burial plots are important to us. They can reflect our personalities and our life values. They are links with our families, past and future. They remind us of our mortality. Yet they are not ultimate. Whether carved in the rock or dug among the rockpiles, our tombs become the portals to partnership in the resurrection for those of us who believe.

"Are Ye Able?" ———————————————

LIKE MOST CANCER PATIENTS, I expect, I've heard my share of "I don't know how you are able to do it!" statements. The person will often go on to say that he or she couldn't bear up so well under the disease. Sometimes I have felt able to bear my cancer, usually when I've been feeling well or when the treatments have been short with few side effects. During these periods having cancer hasn't seemed so devastating. It has been more unpleasant or annoying than disabling and life-threatening. I would just "grin and bear it" until I could get back home, return to teaching, resume my "normal" life. During these times cancer has been a part of my life without yet controlling my life. I could see better days ahead.

Reflecting on these experiences in my own

[99]

life, I remember another of those old hymns from my childhood: "'Are ye able,' said the Master, 'to be crucified with me?' 'Yea,' the sturdy dreamers answered, 'to the death we follow thee.'"* The hymn refers, of course, to Jesus' dialogue with his disciples James and John. Matthew and Mark each contain versions of this exchange. In Mark these two disciples ask a favor of Jesus: "Grant us to sit, one at your right hand and one at your left, in your glory." In reply, Jesus asks, "Are you able to drink the cup that I drink, or to be baptized with the baptism with which I am baptized?" James and John reply, "We are able" (Mark 10:35-39).

I identify with James and John; sometimes I too have felt "able." But these occasions and my confidence haven't lasted. As my disease has progressed, "getting back to normal" has become less and less possible. My own suffering has persuaded me of my inability. Lying in my hospital bed late at night, unable to sleep because of the chemotherapy, my mind races without direction. Here I am not master of my fate. Or again, when I am strapped to a stretcher before lung surgery, I feel helpless. My wife and brother have accom-

* "Are Ye Able," *United Methodist Hymnal* (1989), no. 530.

panied me to the hospital. We have hugged and kissed as I am prepared for surgery. Now they must wait in a distant room as I am wheeled away, first to a waiting area, then down more corridors to an operating room. I am afraid of what the surgery will reveal — but I am even more afraid that I will not wake up afterward.

My earlier ability to handle the situation has been eroded. The cancer seems to be winning. Now I feel more like Peter than like James and John — full of good intentions and false confidence that break down under pressure. After the Last Supper and a walk to the Mount of Olives, Jesus tells his disciples, "You will all fall away . . ." With vigor, we can imagine, Peter fires back his reply to Jesus: "Even though they all fall away, I will not." But Jesus continues, describing how Peter will betray him three times that very night. Still Peter is not shaken. Vehemently he retorts, "If I must die with you, I will not deny you" (Mark 14:26-31). Peter believes that he is ready to die with his Lord. Yet he cannot even keep watch during Jesus' time of prayer in Gethsemane; with James and John, he falls asleep. Even here, with no threats to his own life, "the spirit indeed is willing, but the flesh is weak" (14:32-38). Later that night Peter's betrayal reaches its climax in the courtyard of the high priest. Three times he denies that he has been a disciple of Jesus. And then, when the cock crows twice, Peter remembers Jesus' earlier prediction. Crushed by his own betrayal, "he broke down and wept" (14:66-72).

I can identify with Peter. My intentions to bear my own illness and suffering are good, but my patience and courage often crumble. I cannot comprehend how dying with my cancer can relate to being crucified with Christ. Doubts, frustration, and fear sweep over me. I do not even fully understand Christ's crucifixion. At the conclusion of the passage where James and John seek places of honor, the writer of Mark's Gospel includes these words from Jesus: "For the Son of man also came not to be served but to serve, and to give his life as a ransom for many" (10:45). Is this ransom theology a human attempt to make sense out of Jesus' death? What kind of father would be so immovable as to require a blood sacrifice for the sins of the world and then send his own son to pay that price?

While I do not understand, I find assurance in the action of Jesus, who "came . . . to give his life as a ransom for many." Lying awake at night in the hospital room or strapped to the table before surgery, I am also comforted by Jesus' words. My own inability to understand and to accept my suffering is overcome by Jesus' ability. I am not able to bear up, but God is able. As St. Paul aptly writes, "Likewise the Spirit helps us in our weakness; for we do not know how to pray as we ought, but the Spirit himself intercedes for us with sighs too deep for words" (Rom. 8:26).

Am I able? Not alone. My cancer has knocked me out of the "sturdy dreamers" stage where I could calmly declare with the disciples, "to the death we follow thee." But it has also helped me to discover a higher level of ability.

> Lord, we are able. Our spirits are thine.
> Remold them, make us, like thee, divine.
> Thy guiding radiance above us shall be
> a beacon to God, to love, and loyalty.*

* Ibid.

Christmas:
Joy amidst the Pain ───────────

ON DECEMBER 15 I left my doctor's office at the M.D. Anderson Cancer Center in Houston, Texas. Stepping from the elevator, I walked into the lobby, where I was surprised by singing. Christmas carols resounded through the room. A large crowd surrounded the singers, who were a mixed group of medical center employees. Doctors, nurses, technicians, and others formed the choir. The music continued with gospel songs and "Silent Night" rendered in Spanish. Young and old, men and women, Texan and Mexican, black and white singers blended their enthusiastic voices. I stood at the edge of the crowd, craning to see around the I.V. pole of a patient seated in a wheelchair. As strains of Handel's *Messiah* filled the room, I felt tears well up in my eyes. What a strange place to celebrate Christmas! Looking around, I could see other patients like myself. Intravenous pumps, bandages, or hospital bracelets set us apart. Yet here we were sharing in joyful celebration. We tapped our feet, smiled, and sang along. Somehow the songs raised us above the suffering. We felt joy amidst the pain.

That experience set the tone for my Christmas celebration. I had flown to Texas nine days earlier. My local doctor feared that my cancer had spread to my lungs. I had been coughing and running a fever for weeks. My chest X rays were abnormal. After a night of observation at the local hospital, I caught a flight to Houston the next day. There more tests followed, and more waiting. Finally the announcement: apparently I had only "nonspecific acute and chronic pneumonia." I could fly home tomorrow. With profound relief I telephoned Ruth in North Carolina to share the news. Rarely is the diagnosis of pneumonia greeted with such rejoicing! I would be home for Christmas after all. With this expectation I walked into the lobby filled with carols.

In that lobby, I confronted again the anomaly of my situation. I was filled with excitement and joy over going home; I would make it home to be with Ruth and our sons for Christmas. But in that crowd, amidst the I.V. poles and bandages and my own load of X rays, I couldn't deny the reality of suffering, both my own and that of many around me. I also remembered the call I had received from Ruth two nights before. A beloved member of the congregation had died, another victim of cancer. Joy and pain mixed in that lobby and in my mind.

Flying home on December 16 I had time to meditate. Joy *and* pain — contradictory emotions, they seem; yet they are inextricably linked in my experience of this Christmas. Remembering all of us cancer patients gathered in that lobby, I recognized again that God feels our pain. The celebration there was not simply forgetting our plight; it was experiencing God through it. While I would not profess that God causes our pain so that we will grow in faith, I do believe that suffering becomes an avenue. Along it we can approach the Lord, perhaps more directly than otherwise. Certainly in the Gospel accounts suffering brought many to Christ, the "man full of leprosy" and the woman with "a flow of blood" among many others (Luke 5:12; 8:43). Christ recognized the pain of those who came to him.

In recognizing our pain, God also enables us to celebrate. Often in the Gospels Jesus heals the afflicted, and this healing itself sometimes becomes cause for celebration. For example, the paralytic lowered through the roof takes his bed and goes home, "glorifying God" (Luke 5:25). But even when physical healing does not come, suffering can lead to divine-human encounter. Job provides a classic example. Because of his suffering he approaches God. Job doesn't get the answer he wants; he doesn't hear a justification for his misfortune. But he does now meet God (Job 42:5).

Whether physically restored or not, we are empowered by God to celebrate. I am struck by the short span between Good Friday and Easter in the Christian calendar. Only three days separate the lowest and highest points in Christian experience, from death on the cross to the glory of resurrection. If God heals us, we can celebrate the miracle with the restored paralytic. But in any case, we can pray with Jesus, "Nevertheless not my will, but thine, be done" (Luke 22:42). As I stood in that hospital lobby, I did not know what my future would hold. But I — along with others — was filled with celebration. This, I find, is God with us. At this Christmas season

I can say with that angel who spoke to the shepherds:

> Be not afraid; for behold, I bring you good news
> of a great joy which will come to all the people;
> for to you is born this day in the city of David a
> Savior, who is Christ the Lord. (Luke 2:10-11)

A counterpart to being enabled to celebrate is being empowered to trust God with our destiny. The future is in God's hands. The doctor of internal medicine who directed that medical chorus in the lobby doesn't have all the answers. Something greater than even the cutting edge of medicine was being celebrated there, in the halls of medical science at its best. Something beyond united us all — patients, families, medical staff. Suffering is real, but it is not the final word.

> "Fear not!" said he, for mighty dread
> had seized their troubled mind.
> "Glad tidings of great joy I bring
> to all of humankind . . ."*

* "While Shepherds Watched Their Flocks," *United Methodist Hymnal* (1989), no. 236.

For a few moments on that Friday afternoon in the clinic lobby, the dread lifted from our minds as the modern angels sang. And I recalled again my favorite scripture: "For I am sure that neither death, nor life, . . . nor anything else in all creation, will be able to separate us from the love of God in Christ Jesus our Lord" (Rom. 8:38-39).

Living with Dying: A Daily Endeavor ———————

IN MY EXPERIENCE and that of my family, *living* with dying is perhaps the greatest challenge of my cancer. The hospitalization for chemotherapy, weeks of low blood counts, and periodic CAT scans for re-evaluation come and go. The reports vary, sometimes discouraging, sometimes guardedly optimistic. But through it all, life goes on. Surely death lies before me, somewhere in the distance; "but of that day or that hour no one knows . . ." (Mark 13:32), as Jesus said regarding the end of the age. I am still living now, though the future is unknown.

A good thing that has come out of having cancer is that it has forced me to confront my own finitude. On good days I can sometimes almost forget my cancer, but doctor visits, a nagging cough, or approaching treatment soon jerk me back to reality. I need to be reminded, to keep my life in perspective. So do we all. We are all finite. My family and I have been forced to recognize this more in recent years than ever before.

A central difficulty of living with my illness has been its chronic nature. Unlike some illnesses or conditions, doctors cannot provide a "cure" for my lymphoma. What we have been presented is a series of treatments, more or less effective, designed to control or moderate the cancer's growth. But I was not well prepared for this eventuality. I wanted to hear about cures, not treatments to control. We as a society seem focused on this approach. When something goes wrong, we want it fixed *now* — through surgery, a transplant, or whatever — so that life can return to normal. We are ill prepared for living with chronic illness. My son Eric once commented, "I'd commit suicide if I found out I had cancer." Many would share his perspective.

As I have dealt with my own emotions in response to my illness, I have come to believe that dying itself may be easier than living with dying. The event of death is relatively brief, but the process of dying can stretch across years.

When you *know* you are dying, your mechanisms of denial are much less effective. No wonder many young people say they would prefer to die quickly of a heart attack. Such a death avoids the wrestling with one's finitude which accompanies chronic illness. With chronic illness, the pain, depression, and disability may be endured for years. Here there is no sharp dividing line between living and dying. Instead, we enter the gray area of living with dying. Death is an unavoidable presence, yet so is life.

Reading the Gospels from the perspective of my own struggle to live with dying, I am struck by Jesus' creative living in the shadow of the cross. In the very center of Mark's Gospel, Jesus tells his disciples about his own approaching death:

> And he began to teach them that the Son of man must suffer many things, and be rejected by the elders and the chief priests and the scribes, and be killed, and after three days rise again. (8:31)

As we have seen, Peter immediately rebukes Jesus. Peter was like us. He was not yet ready for Jesus to die, nor was he ready to die himself.

But how does Jesus respond to the knowledge

of his own approaching death? The second half of Mark's Gospel reveals how he lives his remaining days. Jesus continues the ministry of preaching, teaching, healing, and casting out demons which he has begun. Here we see the concern for the spiritually and physically needy which typifies his entire ministry. In addition, Jesus continues to train his disciples, now injecting the new elements of his approaching death and the necessity of suffering in their own lives (Mark 8:31, 34-35). Throughout these endeavors Jesus appears remarkably free of self-pity. Still, he too experiences the human will to live. In the garden with Peter, James, and John, he "began to be greatly distressed and troubled." He then reports to the disciples, "My soul is very sorrowful, even to death" (14:33, 34). His prayer in Gethsemane reveals his honest desire to continue living, to finish his work, yet he subdues his own will to God's will (14:36). Here may lie the clue to his overall attitude. In the Gospel accounts, Jesus emerges as convinced that his death is God's will, but even more, that he can trust his life and death to God. In his first words to the disciples about his eventual death, Jesus concludes by reporting that after three days he will rise again (8:31). God will prevail, even over death. There in the garden, Jesus ends his prayer, "Yet not what I will, but what thou wilt" (14:36).

From reflections upon Jesus' living with dying, I return to my own situation. What perspective have I gained? Above all, I find, is one's relationship to God. Can we trust God with our destiny, even in death? Can we also surrender our living to God? This theology of surrender which I described at the beginning of these reflections provides the foundation for living with dying. If we find God trustworthy, not only dying but also living with dying becomes possible, as it was for Jesus. The Lord indeed becomes our shepherd who leads us and restores our souls.

From this foundation new possibilities emerge. One discovery which I have made is that the suffering of illness and treatment can become a hurdle to be crossed, rather than a wall blocking my way. Jesus' knowledge of his approaching death did not stop his ministry. Chronic illness need not completely shut us off from living either. The suffering is real, but much can be overcome if we are not engulfed by the pain at hand. The chemotherapy, the surgery, and the pneumonia become hurdles which we must cross in living with dying. Each procedure in itself is not a wall but a hurdle along one's path. In viewing suffering as a hurdle I have found much strength and energy to pursue the living which remains.

Another perspective emerging from my experience is that of focusing upon each day, one at a time. Ruth distilled the essence of our family's orientation when she said, "I have to decide again every day whether you're living or dying." While this may sound callous, it captures the truth that the balance between living and dying fluctuates with an illness like my cancer. When chemotherapy or complications confront us, dying is at the forefront. Between treatments, when I am feeling well, living takes first place. Neither ever completely dispels the other. Thus we are living with dying. But the focus of the day depends upon which is now before us.

This shifting focus points to another dimension of our experience: seeking to live fully in the present. As I've described earlier, the future is uncertain, but the present is ours, as a gift. More than ever, I am learning to live, to enjoy life now. To be thankful for what strength I have, for material blessings, for people I love. Perhaps partly because of middle age, more because of my illness, I have come to a greater appreciation of where I am and focus less upon distant future goals. To recall Jesus' words again, no one knows the day or the hour. But I do have the present to live.

This living in the present requires flexibility, however. I've described elsewhere the inability to plan that is a part of living with chronic illness. My family has learned the hard way that flexibility needs to be built into our lives. This flexibility does not mean that all plans are thrown aside, but it does suggest that plans become tentative and that one must be honest with others about the nature of these commitments. This shift in orientation can be very difficult for those of us who have sought to be people of our word, persons who never let others down. My illness has placed particular burdens upon Ruth in this regard, as she has sought to juggle children, her job, and my illness. But flexibility has enabled us to follow plans when possible and to change them as necessary. Gradually, too, we have sensed some lessening of guilt over our undependability.

Through living with dying I have also discovered afresh the meaning and importance of relationships. Confronted with my own finitude, I appreciate more than ever my relationship with my wife. I realize how much her own sacrifice has meant in strengthening me in my struggle. I also have spent more time with my sons, listening to them and doing with them the activities that they enjoy. Being a strong father for them now, I believe, may be my greatest legacy to them. Relationships with friends outside the family circle have also gained new significance. The love and tangible support of many have taught me more clearly that we do not die — or live — completely alone.

My struggle with cancer, then, has been a daily endeavor of living with dying. I continue on with the help of past experiences, through the strength of others, and in the presence of Christ. Now as never before, Paul's words in Romans speak boldly to me:

If we live, we live to the Lord,
and if we die, we die to the Lord;
so then, whether we live or whether we die,
we are the Lord's.
(Rom. 14:8, emphasis added)